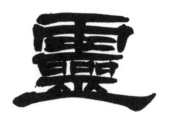

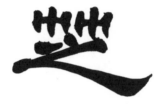

Reishi Mushroom

Herb of Spiritual Potency
and Medical Wonder

"They dose themselves with the germ of gold and jade,
eat the finest fruit of the purple polypore fungus.
By eating what is germinal their bodies are lightened,
and so they are capable of spiritual transcendence."

First century philosopher Wang Ch'ung, describing Taoist practices.
Time-Life Books, Great Ages of Man: Ancient China.

REISHI MUSHROOM

Herb of Spiritual Potency
and
Medical Wonder

by
Terry Willard, Ph.D.

Research by Kenneth Jones

Sylvan Press
Issaquah, Washington

ISBN: 0-9625638-0-3

Published by Sylvan Press
1420 Gilman Blvd. Suite 2265
Issaquah, Washington 98207

Layout by James McCormick
Cover Design by Francine Katz

Printed in Hong Kong

Acknowledgements

Working on a book requires the contributions of many people. This book represents the collected feedback and thought-provoking discussions I have had with dozens of scientists, researchers, patients, students and doctors. Stretching over eighteen months, we communicated in print, by fax and via phone.

Many of these people appear throughout the text but some remain anonymous or unrecognized. Some are people who stimulated my interest, an herb merchant in Hong Kong, for example. Others led me to examine my own ideas on health care, voices without names who asked questions about the immune system during phone-in talk shows. Thankfully there are a handful of people who can be identified. They had very direct effect on this work.

The concepts outlined by Dr. Wu of Shanghai sparked this project initially. The outstanding research efforts of Ken Jones made it possible to work through all the materials despite my busy schedule. Without his input, this project could never have been completed.

Support from mycologist Jeff Chilton, both editorial and scientific, put the project on a more solid basis. Additional taxonomic assistance by Ruey Shyang Hseu is greatly appreciated. Norm and Natsuko Goundry made an invaluable contribution by translating works in Japanese and perplexing medieval Chinese.

As with my two previous books, James McCormick, M.Sc. provided editorial assistance. His creativity and organizational skill helped to finish this project in such a short time. The publisher, Fred Katz, contributed a great deal through a constructively critical reading of the manuscript. Fred's comments lent greater clarity to the text. The book cover was artfully designed by Francine Katz.

I would like to thank the following people for their excellent photographs and photographic contributions: Hajo Hadeler, Francine Katz, J.S. Chilton, Ruey-Shyang Hseu, J.H. Petersen, Coleman Luthie, Blaine Andrusek and Canited International Ltd. Dr. David Chu kindly provided the calligraphy for the word *Ling zhi*.

The direct feedback of many holistic health colleagues should be noted: Paul Lee, Michael Broffman, Andrew Weil, Subhuti Dharman-anda, David Chu, Bill Brevoort, Mark Blumenthal, Paul Larsen, and Rob McCaleb all contributed their knowledge and experiences with Reishi.

To all of these people I am deeply indebted for their commitment to the completion of the manuscript in spite of everyone's other responsibilities. Writing this book has made me keenly aware of the excitement of learning and our need to explore the frontiers of herbal knowledge.

Calgary, Spring 1990

FOREWORD

It is my pleasure to introduce this book about one of the most important medicinal plants of the age—the magic Reishi mushroom, or Ling zhi as it is called in China. To introduce Reishi to a wide audience, it is the challenging job of the author, Terry Willard, to overcome two cultural factors: a cultural bias and a cultural amnesia. I believe he is up to the task.

Why cultural bias? In North America, it is common to observe a rather strong "mycophobia," or fear of mushrooms. It seems to be mainly from the British that we inherited this fear, as is apparent to anyone reading the line from the great English writer Sir Arthur Conan Doyle (author of Sherlock Holmes), that mushrooms "like foul postules from the earth..." sprung up after a rain. This description paints a rather unsavory picture of the whole fungal kingdom. But are these interesting creations really so bad? Most cultures of the world feel quite the opposite!

Fortunately, in North America we have a very diverse cultural mix, perhaps helping us to avoid completely closing our minds to new things. It is a fact that most cultures, rather than detesting mushrooms, not only love them, but ardently seek them for both food and medicine. In fact, they gladly pay high prices for them. In Russia, all over Europe, and across the Orient, people are mad over mushrooms. For instance, in Japan, collectors go into the hills and gather particular kinds of medicinal fungi called polypores, returning to town to sell them on the streets in push-carts. These invigorating and therapeutic magical mushrooms are eagerly purchased, to be taken home and added to soups, stews and teas.

Wherein lies the cultural amnesia of which I spoke? We have forgotten about the concept of "tonics," and we are only just now re-focusing our attention on the idea of health preservation through prevention. A tonic in the present sense is a natural substance that generally strengthens and supports body systems. This concept is a vital one, for in this age, where environmental conditions are rapidly changing, our food, water, and even the very air we breathe are being polluted with the addition of many new synthetic chemical compounds. These compounds, in addition to the stressors of fast-paced life-styles, the pressure of increased population, the weakening of the protective ozone layer, and other novel strains on our immune system, make it easy to understand the desirability of natural products that can strengthen our defense systems and act as general environmental safeguards.

Reishi is one of the foremost of these natural products. In fact, there are other "medicinal mushrooms" such as Shiitake, *Coriolus versicolor*, and *Schizophyllum commune*, that show great promise, but Reishi is one of the ancient ones—with not only a long history (thousands of years) of safe use, but also an incredible array of modern scientific "provings" in both the laboratory and the clinic.

I have observed that some people, when considering Reishi as part of a strengthening program with other herbal remedies for their immune system, invariably ask the question: "But if I have an allergy to fungi, how can I take Reishi?" Through 15 years of personal experience with medicinal mushrooms—wandering through the woods eating them, brewing mushroom elixirs, sifting through the scientific literature and recommending them in my herbal practice—I have never read about or observed anyone having an allergic reaction to them, no matter how sensitive to moulds, or how severe a case of "candidiasis" they believe they may have. In fact, I have often seen these mushrooms support and re-balance the defensive and vital energy of the body.

People also ask how often to take Reishi as a medicine. Another way of looking at the whole process is the view of not only the Chinese healer, but also of Hippocrates, the ancient Nature-Doctor who said: "let your medicine be your food and your food be your medicine." Consider Reishi a food—one to be eaten often, when needed for strengthening and "environmental protection." In this way we embrace the concept of tonics—natural food-medicines which can nourish and strengthen us. In this culture, we are not unfamiliar with this concept as seen, for instance, in advertising for milk. These ads extol the "healthful" virtues of milk, telling us in particular that it helps build "strong bones." Recognize that Reishi and other adaptogens help us build strong defenses.

In summary, I believe you will find Terry Willard's book not only absorbing, but of importance in re-emphasizing an age-old approach to health and prevention. He has presented the material in a style that involves us in a adventure of discovery, and helps to make the scientific provings more accessible. I hope my short introduction not only serves to open the door to the exciting work in your hands, but also helps to impart a little of the love and tremendous enthusiasm I have for medicinal mushrooms and our future relationship with them.

Christopher Hobbs
Santa Cruz, CA.
April 14, 1990

Table of Contents

List of Illustrations

Introduction

T he crowded bustling street of Hong Kong might seem an unlikely place for a Canadian herbalist to start a story. But in 1987 I found myself looking through a small storefront window at the paraphernalia of Oriental herbalism.

The long pale roots of the famous ginseng sat with prices as high as $100,000. Exotic substances like antler horn and special pearls were displayed with all the pomp and circumstance of jewelry. Dried herbs and jars of powder lay on shelves amid brightly coloured bottles of patent medicine. Row upon row of dark mahogany boxes lay behind the long wooden dispensing table, filled with substances that I could only guess about.

What caught my attention that day was a mushroom. More precisely it was a wooden mushroom. There it stood, in the position of honour in the little shop. I was puzzled.

For several years I had read about Shiitake (pronounced SHE-tah-key), a mushroom used in many Oriental dishes. I had eaten it enthusiastically at sushi bars (a favourite pastime of mine). So when I went into the small aromatic store I assumed this was some sort of statue venerating Shiitake's health benefits.

But when I used sign language to communicate with the Cantonese herbalist, it was clear the mushroom statue was in fact the mushroom itself. And even with my very, very limited Chinese, I could tell that its name didn't remotely resemble Shiitake.

An herbal mystery was left unsolved that day. Through a series of unlikely events I was going to learn a lot more about the "wooden mushroom." It was the start of an adventure that would lead from Shanghai to the coast of British Columbia, from the work of a giant Japanese corporation to the diligence of a few men living in a small Canadian town. The trail would lead me from San Francisco through Southern California and would persuade me to learn a great deal more about an herb that was to have a significant influence on my own life and that of my patients.

Over and over, the mushroom reappeared in my life, in conversations, in chance encounters and ultimately as part of my professional life.

1

Its name is *Reishi* (or *Ling zhi*) and it has had a treasured role in the Orient for centuries. Now an object of scientific research, Reishi is poised for popularity around the world. And with the mushroom now cultivated, rather than painstakingly gleaned from distant forests, many more people will benefit from Reishi than in the past.

My involvement with Reishi leads back to my decision to become an herbalist.

In the early 1970s I was a university student registered in Environmental Biology at the University of Calgary. As many people around the world found out during the 1988 Winter Olympics, Calgary is rather unusual. A city of 600,000 people, it sits on the edge of prairie and mountain—a mere 45 minutes by car from the haunts of grizzly bears, mountain goats and cougar.

Through simple good fortune, a summer job took me to a high alpine valley in the Canadian Rockies. My task was to study the effects of forest fires on the rugged terrain and the plant life. That summer was to have a profound effect on the course of my life.

Day after day I traipsed over the rugged ground, applying the arcane methods which biologists use to study plant distribution. Amidst the careful records and routines of biological science I was struck by the wealth of plants, even in an environment where the harsh winter storms were matched only by the beautiful sunlit summers.

Week followed week and my knowledge about the environment deepened. I knew the following plants by sight: Fireweed, Horsetail, Fleabane, Woundwort, Indian Paintbrush, Biscuitroot, Bearberry and Lungwort.

These names spoke of a history that I knew nothing about. Where did the names come from? Did fleabane or woundwort really work as their names suggested? By the end of the summer I was looking forward to returning to university where I might find books or articles which would answer my questions about this abundant plantlife.

When I returned to university that fall, one of my professors, Steve Herrero, allowed me to conduct a personal research project on the edible and medicinal attributes of the Alberta Rocky Mountain plants I had studied more "scientifically" during the summer.

The project was to open my eyes. I had been vaguely aware of the value of plants as foods and medicines but I hadn't realized that the mountains surrounding the city of Calgary contained a complete pharmacopoeia and food source. Both Native Americans and European pioneers had depended on these resources for their very lives.

Well before the appearance of doctors in the Canadian West, herbalists and 'root doctors' plied a trade, calming fevers, setting bones, easing arthritis and providing health care at its most basic level. And

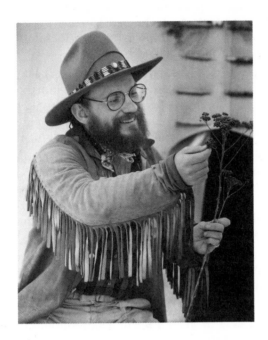

The author studying an herb in front of his tipi

before them the native peoples of the region had centuries to observe the plant and animal life of the country and put it to use. The native shamans were driven out and persecuted when the white people came. Today we see a resurgence of native healing and native healing methods, even in the hospitals of modern Canada.

First Steps in Herbalism

As I studied the medical history of the Rocky Mountain plants, I became more and more enthusiastic about their properties. Like every "convert," I never hesitated to bend someone's ear when it came time to talk about my interests. As people came to know me as the "herb guy," they started to ask me for more specific information on how to use herbs. Between my studies and the questions of others, I started to experiment with plants as a means of simple first-aid and health improvement.

As time passed, my enthusiasm grew and herbs became a dominant force in my life. Rather effortlessly I became a novice herbalist. The university took some notice and I was asked to teach an extension course on the edible and medicinal properties of the Rocky Mountain plants.

When I completed my Bachelor of Science degree, I found myself at loose ends. I considered applying for medical school but realized that the knowledge about the natural world which I had worked to collect was all but ignored by modern medicine. I had a decision to make and ultimately decided to become a professional herbalist, to seek the training wherever it could be found and to combine my scientific training with the real health benefits of the plants that surround us.

The best place for me to start was in my own backyard. I bought a tipi and went up to the mountains to live like an Indian. At that point in my life I was a vegetarian and decided to eat only wild plants. It wasn't long before I learned all the edible plants within walking distance of my tipi. I found myself spending many hours a day "grazing."

As winter approached I decided I could weather the -45° temperatures in a tipi, but to do this I'd need to join with other people. As winter set in, a small group of like-minded people set up camp on North Burnt Timber Creek. It was surprisingly easy to acclimatize to the cooler weather, especially after others in camp convinced me that deer meat was not all that bad for humans.

I spent the next two years learning from the Indians while gleaning anything I could on herbs from written accounts. At this point in time I met a very charismatic man, Dr. J.R. Christopher, who possessed a tremendous knowledge of herbs.

Over the next few years I spent a fair amount of time with Dr. Christopher and eventually helped him with his burden of lecture tours that he conducted for the Nature's Way herb company. As he grew older and less able to keep up the hectic touring pace, I had the chance to travel all over North America lecturing in his place. Throughout this period, I had a chance to study with other well-known natural healers, such as Dr. Bernard Jensen (Iridology) in southern California and Frater Albertus (Western alchemy) at his Paracelsus mountain retreat.

When not travelling to lecture or study, I began consulting with the public on the use of herbs. My small consulting business grew into a series of courses on herbology and iridology. In 1975 I incorporated the Wild Rose College of Natural Healing. In subsequent years, Wild Rose was responsible for introducing hundreds of people to concepts of herbalism and alternative medicine. Our curriculum branched out to offer diploma programs, weekend seminars and intensive research projects. With classroom courses in Calgary and Vancouver and correspondence students scattered around the world, the college has been a major part of my life. So much so that my own education has often been wedged into small parts of a busy schedule.

Through the early 1980s the Wild Rose College of Natural Healing continued to grow and the herbology course grew from a set of handouts to a set of heavy manuals. By the mid-'80s there was a line of Wild Rose herbal formulas, clinics and classrooms in Vancouver and Calgary, regular trips to conventions, lecture tours and the publication of two books.

As herbs started to gain respectability in the 80s, the health food market began to pay greater attention to Oriental herbs. My own research kept uncovering their benefits and eventually I was able to integrate these herbs into my formulas and consulting practice.

With my growing appetite for learning about Oriental healing and culture, it wasn't long before I was planning to visit the Orient. Trips to the Philippines, Hong Kong, Thailand and Bali became working vacations. I met herbalists everywhere I went.

And that is what brought me to the small herb shop on a side-street in Hong Kong.

Chapter 1
The Emperor's Search:
The Folklore of Reishi

The mystery and folklore surrounding Reishi extends back through the ancient history of China, but my first real exposure was in the very modern Sheraton hotel in bustling Shanghai.

Entering the Sheraton's premier restaurant, the first thing that greets you is a gnarled and strangely beautiful 200 year old bonsai. It stood as the focal point in the foyer on the top of the Hua Ting Shanghai Sheraton. A question immediately popped into my head. How could such a rugged yet delicate tree live in three inches of soil?

The surroundings in this eagle's perch overlooking the city wer lavish in comparison to the day to day realities for most of Shanghai's million people. Lightly lacquered wood, blond instead of the norm deep mahogany, was everywhere in evidence. The attractive hostess w dressed in traditional Chinese court garb. This restaurant was suppos to be one of the best in the city of adventurous mysteries—*Pu chiang*

I wanted very much to impress my guest, Dr. Wu. He was wic considered to be one of the authorities on medicinal plants, speciali in *Fu Zheng* (pronounced FOO-shen) therapy, a subject I was anxio learn more about. He was also well-known for his love of the del tastes that can only come from the kitchens of great Oriental master

Dr. Wu had met me in the main lobby and after coming up the elevator we now stood in a small lobby on the top floor.

"Doctor Willard?" the hostess said. After identifying mys directed us to our seats overlooking Shanghai. We both commer the luck of facing west to be able to see the sunset. Luck was also side because Dr. Wu's English was so clear. The meal wou affected by the slow and sometimes strained use of translators.

I was on a six-week tour of China to learn more about the tr medicine based on botanicals. It was a system that had surviv 5,000 years and though quite different from Western scientific it still retained an undeniable vigour and intellectual cohesiv theory behind the medicine had undergone evolution and decay through the centuries, yet it was still effective enough that hundreds of millions of people around the world considered it their primary form of health-care.

If statistics are important, traditional Chinese medicine has them in spades. It has effectively treated billions of people over thousands of years. At first glance Westerners might find it archaic. For instance, Oriental medicine uses more natural categories for defining states of health and the surrounding environment. The practical research of Oriental doctors through the centuries holds hope for some of North America's greatest health problems. My main interest was possible herbal solutions to the growing "attack" on the immune system by the many diseases which were baffling Western medical researchers.

I started my journey as a People to People delegate on an herbal medicine trade delegation. A group of 10 scholars, herbalists and herb producers had travelled together for two weeks. I was now on my own. I had already been in China for three weeks, spending time in Beijing, Chendu, Shanghai, Guanjhou and Hong Kong. I was getting more accustomed to the Chinese way of doing things. Though I had travelled through southeast Asia before, this was my first trip to the mainland and it seemed like another world entirely.

I felt comfortable returning to Shanghai as a solitary traveller, the city that seemed most promising for my investigations. Through a passing scholar, I had heard a little about a certain Doctor Wu, an expert on a traditional form of immunotherapy called *Fu Zheng* therapy. But nothing could have prepared me for the next several hours.

Although I was the official host, having invited Dr. Wu, I immediately deferred the selection of dishes to him. As a connoisseur of Chinese teas, Dr. Wu said that the most important aspect of the whole meal was the tea. "Once the flavour of the tea was established, then the palate will immediately lead us to the rest of the menu." Dr. Wu's brief burst of Chinese to the waiter brought a menu. But it was a menu which listed only teas.

Understandably, Dr. Wu considered the choice of a fine tea to be beyond the competence of a mere *Kwei low* (foreign devil), but I was a bit surprised that his appreciation for tea was matched by the restaurant's selection. The tea menu itself was four pages long!

There were two pages assigned to green tea and two pages to red tea (which we would call black tea). Was this any different than a fine French restaurant which would offer pages of white and red wines? I was asked if I preferred red or green tea. Through experience I knew the green was best for me and fortunately Dr. Wu was amenable. He began to read through the choices of green tea.

"Being summer, it has been very hot lately," Dr. Wu stated. A modest understatement, I thought, since the temperature outside was 110 degrees Fahrenheit. Being from the Canadian prairies, I wasn't prepared for the extreme heat and humidity at sea level in a foreign country. Dr. Wu announced, "We should drink *Zhong Guo Ming Cha*. This tea is made from specially picked spring blossoms of the tea plant, only found in the Black Dragon Spring Hills near Haunzhou. Past emperors travelled there in the summer to drink this tea, as it is known to cool down the inside temperature of a person in the summer."

After taking two showers a day to cool myself down, I was all for that. Any break from the heat would be welcome. "That sounds good to me", I said, doing my best to cover my relief.

Dinner was then ordered and the tea arrived. It was served a little differently than normal. Instead of bringing a tea pot for the tea to steep in, a small amount was placed in our porcelain mugs, hot water was poured over it and a lid was put on top. My immediate thought was, "how is a hot tea going to cool me down?" but I kept my mouth shut and waited to see what would happen.

Dr. Wu said, "This is one of the most expensive teas in China, about $35.00 per kilo, but it goes a long way. The first cup is not the best. You should only drink about two-thirds of the cup and fill it with more water. With wine, the first drops are the best but with tea the last are the best." I tapped the table with my fingertips as the waiter poured the tea water. Dr. Wu looked at me and laughed, "So you have been to southern China, I see.

"Do you know the origin of tapping the fingers on the dinner table in thanks for someone pouring tea?" he asked.

I shook my head. "It's just a habit I picked up from Chinese friends," I said.

We took a sip of excellent tea and Dr. Wu began a story.

"In the past, emperors had a very hard time travelling. For them to travel a mere seven miles from the Forbidden City to the Summer Palace required an entourage of 150,000 and a trip in night time. It was against the law for a mere mortal Chinese to see the Emperor, the direct descendant of the Gods. In the 18th century one Emperor decided to travel this seven miles during the day. For this they constructed a silk tunnel seven miles long, wide enough for 50 people walking side by side. One account suggested that this tunnel required more silk than had ever been sold to the West up to that time.

"In this atmosphere it was impossible for the Emperor to travel China and see the countryside as a normal person would. One Emperor did travel as a peasant in southern China accompanied only by his bodyguards. Upon entering an inn for dinner, a tea pot was placed in front of him. Protocol dictated that he must pour the tea for the others. Rather than risk detection he poured tea for his bodyguards. A rather unthinkable breech of tradition!

"Protocol also stated that all imperial subjects had to kowtow — a very deep bow — when the Emperor was present or had performed even a slight action. To fail to do so could mean decapitation.

"Shock and confusion reigned amongst the Emperor's guards for a moment until one of them quick-wittedly placed his ring and first finger on the dinner table and made a symbolic kowtow with his index finger. Thus the kowtow could be performed without revealing the Emperor's identity.

"And ever since, in the Canton Province of China, moving the fingers thus has been a method of showing respect for a tea pourer. Some say that it also shows you are enjoying the food so much that your mouth is full. Rather than neglect to thank the tea pourer or impolitely speak with one's mouth full, one performs the finger tap gesture — a less exotic story but one full of logic."

We continued to drink our tea and make small talk about how I liked China, what kind of things I did in Canada and other bits of trivia until our food came. Each dish seemed to taste better than the one before. I was in heaven. There was no doubt in my mind that good Chinese food, cooked in the right way, is some of the best food in the world.

As the dinner drew to its conclusion I decided it was time to ask my questions. I didn't want him to simply get up and leave, as is all too often the case with mainland Chinese.

I told him I was very interested in herbs that would build up the body-protection system, herbs that would enhance the immune system and possibly reverse degeneration. I was interested in his ideas on diseases such as AIDS, Epstein-Barr virus (EBV) or Chronic Fatigue syndrome (CFS). I had heard of *Fu Zheng* therapy and was interested in learning more. I knew that *Astragalus* and *Ligustrum lucidum* were both used in *Fu Zheng*, but there must be more.

I told him that I had formulated products in Canada that combined *Astragalus* (*Huang qi*), Licorice (*Gan-cao*) and a North American Indian plant, Echinacea. I had been having great success with this product for colds, sore throats, and (when used with *Beta*-carotene) for building up thymic function.

Dr. Wu said, "Well, *Huang qi*, *Ligustrum* and *Gan-cao* were all good *Fu Zheng* herbs, but they are of small value compared to *Ling zhi*."

Ling zhi . . . I knew I had heard of it somewhere, but what was it? I told him I was only a little bit familiar with the name and couldn't place it. As he described the plant, my mind immediately jumped back to the herb store in Hong Kong that I had visited a year earlier — to the mushroom I had mistaken for a statue venerating Shiitake. *Ling zhi* was what the Japanese call Reishi.(pronounced REE-she.)

I told Dr. Wu I had seen Reishi before and that I was all ears. I told him about seeing it in Korea in a place of great importance in the herbalist's shop.

Where does it come from and if it is so special, why don't we see it in common herbal formulas made from Chinese herbs?" I asked.

"Well, it has been a great secret and a rare plant. It was revered by the old Taoists, you know," replied Dr. Wu.

Now I became very interested. One of my favourite pastimes was to read accounts of the alchemy of the ancient Taoists. Alchemy involved the search for miraculous medicines, life-enhancing substances and the ability to turn base metals into gold.

I told him I had a little familiarity with Taoist ideas, though only from a Western point of view. I had read a few translations of *Tao teh Ching* and *Hua Hu Ching* by Lao Tzu and was quite fascinated by these concepts.

Dr. Wu started, "Well, the Taoists are the source of much of our modern Chinese medicine. The Taoists believe in immortality. Their goal was to flow into the great Tao and become one of the immortals, joining the constellation. In the pursuit of this they practised many strange arts, one of which was the careful search for the elixir of life.

"Many feel that the *Ling zhi*, or should I call it Reishi, as it is the name you are familiar with, was a major ingredient of this great elixir if not the elixir of immortality itself."

Anyone in the restaurant that evening who happened to look my way at that moment would have seen me wide-eyed, probably with my chin hitting my knees. I was certainly enjoying the story and Dr. Wu knew it. So he went on.

"In Chinese the word *Ling* is composed of the pictures for *rain, shaman*, and *praying for,* together meaning *spiritual potency, or a stirring of the soul. Chih* means tree fungus and substances used to concoct elixirs of immortality. Thus the `herb of spiritual potency.'

"In the 3rd century B.C., China was shrouded in an atmosphere of magic. To the uninitiated, the concept of a miracle-cure for mortality had become nothing short of a cult. One purveyor of medicine, a master An-Chi, was said by people to be over a century old. Later accounts refer to him as an immortal.

"Along the shore at Fou-hsing, a place not far from the present city of Tsingtao, where the beer comes from, in the Province of Shandong, China's self-proclaimed First Emperor, Shih Huang Ti (BC 259-210), the Yellow Emperor, whose Great Wall stands even today, had many temples erected to the immortals in an effort to lure those with knowledge of manufacturing elixirs. During his time, stories were circulating that living on some mountainous isles out to sea were not one but many

11

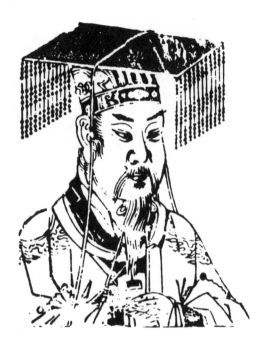

The First Emperor of China, Chin Shih Huang Ti

immortals and nearby, the `herb of deathlessness', a magical mushroom (*chih*). Should it be eaten, one would immediately attain long life and immortality.

"An official report related that such a plant was seen held in the beaks of raven-like birds that flew to the site of a massacre in the far western reaches of the empire at Ferghana. They had placed the plant on the dead men's faces, whereupon the corpses `immediately sat up and were restored to life.'

"Receiving this extraordinary report from the officials, along with a small sample of the herb, the Emperor quickly dispatched an envoy to have it identified by Kuei Ku hsien-seng, or `Devil-Valley Master,' who lived to the north of the city. He recognized it at once. It was indeed the `herb of deathlessness,' the same one that grew among rose-coloured rocks in fields on the isle of Tsu-Chou. A single stalk would suffice to bring a dead man back to life. He added, it was also known as `the (magic) mushroom that nourishes the spirit (*yang shen chih*).'

"The Emperor was of course thrilled and with a Taoist named Hsu Fu as admiral, in B.C. 219 he dispatched a whole fleet of ships and 500 young subjects (250 girls and 250 boys) to sail to the east and not come back till they found the mushroom or herb of deathlessness.

"One account says that Admiral Hsu Fu never returned. Another recounts that Hsu Fu sailed with 3,000 youths, maidens and labourers. After reaching their destination Hsu Fu proclaimed himself king. Many believe that the destination was Japan. To this day, near the city of Shingu in Wakayama, lies the grave of a great alchemist named Hsu Fu, a pilgrimage site for the ill."

At this time more hot water was poured into the tea and a natural pause occurred.

"Did Shih Huang Ti ever find the mushroom and use it?" I asked.

"Well, that is the interesting part," replied Dr. Wu. "Shih Huang Ti was so obsessed with this elixir and longevity that it finally became his downfall. The Emperor had decided that all knowledge was going to start with him, so he burned all of the books in the empire, rewriting the ones he wanted.

"In some of the most secret books were versions of the elixir's formula. The formula called for the use of large amounts of mercury, to make the big red pill of immortality. Though not sure of the exact formula (because of the destruction of all books), the Emperor decreed that the pill be concocted. The mercury was to increase the power of *Sheng Qi* (the spirit energy). The problem of course is that mercury is extremely toxic.

"After the *Sheng Qi* was caused to burn brighter and stronger, the toxic effect would kill a person. At this stage a specific formula based on a unique shape of *Ling zhi* was given to stop the rage of the poison while keeping the *Sheng Qi* burning bright to bring about the state of longevity.

"It appears that Shih Huang Ti either didn't have the formula right or he didn't get the right *Ling zhi* in time. We do know he sent many servants up into the mountains to find it and that he himself ventured out to find it. Ultimately, he died in his own litter, searching for this elixir for mercury poisoning.

"In this ancient quest for an elixir of longevity, there were five kinds of *Chih*: Stone *chih*, grass *chih*, wood *chih*, flesh *chih* and mushroom *chih*. Of the mushroom *chih* there were supposed to be 120 kinds of these substances. They ranged in potency, producing a short longevity of 100 years, up to the potent forms which ensured a life of over 1,000 years.

"The *chun-chih* or 'mushroom chih' is referred to in the singular tense as if there is only one species of mushroom that grows deep in the mountains, usually under big trees or beside springs. The Taoists say the *chun-chih* is reminiscent of the human body, a palace, flying birds, a tiger, a coach horse or a dragon.

"It is also known to come in any one of six colors: red, yellow, black, white, green or blue. The red is the strongest and ingesting 'a square inch' of a properly shaped *chun-chih* would cause one to 'rise up to the immortals.'"

13

However steeped in metaphor to confound the uninitiated, this was starting to sound like the mushrooms consumed during the hippie era in North America — psychedelic mushrooms — so I mentioned it. Dr. Wu said that this mushroom did not have psychotropic properties, just spiritual potency.

"Looking at the old Taoist writings and art we can tell to a certain degree that this is the mushroom you call Reishi," he continued. "It is said to grow on Mount Heng-shan in Hunan Province. It tasted bitter, like Reishi, and was non-poisonous, like many of the psychotropic mushrooms.

"This is not to say that no Taoists tried psychotropic mushrooms in order to find the elixir of the gods, as one can understand that both in the West and the East many alchemists died prematurely in the pursuit of immortality. Because the most potent Reishi is considered to be the red one, probably many took *Amanita muscaria* and got poisoned. But the ancients did leave plenty of pictures of a Taoist carrying the mushroom of immortality, placing it in the Taoist mountains and portraying it as the *hsien-shen* drug among the drugs of immortality.

"Ko Hung, a Taoist and one of the great alchemist-physicians, lived from A.D. 281 to 361. He stated that the *chih* plant could ward off evil and grew in five suitable mountains corresponding to the Taoist's five sacred mountains. Today Reishi can be harvested on one of these mountains, Mount Tai-shan, located in Shangdong Province.

"Ko Hung's written works continuously refer to *The Four Canons of Shen-nung*. Shen-nung lived B.C. 2838 and is believed to be the inventor of medicine and agriculture. In his work he graded medicines according to three functional classes: superior, inferior and medium quality. The mushroom was classified as the top of the superior quality.

"The ancients preferred the tougher Polypores to normal mushrooms, originally giving them the name *ch'i* (now spelled *qi*). But the word *ch'i* has more conspicuous meanings to the Taoist, such as *prime matter* or *One soul, Ik-ch'i* --a primordial entity, `*self-expanding as vapour.*' To the alchemists, the Prime Matter was an *immortal substance* synonymous with *elixir*. This elixir was not meant to be a mere tonic. It was to vivify the entire system and to impart `immortality.' This *qi* plant is also found in India as an elixir.

"To the ancients, red, as the color of blood, equated with *Soul*, and anything in Nature so-signatured became accordingly auspicious as an embodiment of *ch'i* or Soul. Because of this, the potency of the medicine, be it herbal or mineral, was the amount of Soul it held.

"The word *chih* also means red, which is probably why the red Reishi is considered the strongest. One thing is certain. The *Chih* mushroom is conspicuous in the earliest records of alchemy in China. For these reasons it is easy to see why *Ling zhi* or *Reishi*, the spiritual fungus, has often been treasured more than gold."

Sipping on the refreshing tea, I wondered if any of these myths could be true. Was Dr. Wu just stringing along a gullible Westerner? I asked him, "Is there any solid evidence to link modern day Reishi to this ancient mushroom of immortality?"

"Oh yes," he responded. "The *chih* mushroom appears in the medical literature of every dynasty in China. We can say that no work is as comprehensive as that finished in 1578 during the Ming Dynasty, when the physician Li Shih-chen spent 26 years compiling the then known records of Chinese medicine. He published the *Pen T'sao Kang Mu (or Ben Cao Gang Mu)* — The Great Pharmacopoeia.

"These works identify Reishi as the *Chi zhi* or `red fungus,' then also being called *Dan zhi* or the `Red Pill fungus', an herb of the immortals. It is this fungus that corresponds with the mushroom we call today *Ling zhi*. The ancient Taoists specified the Red Chi or *ch'i chi* (ch'i fungus), which they also called `cinnabar' chi *(tan chi)*. It grew on Mount Heng-shan in Hunan Province, the southern site of the Taoist's five sacred mountains. Like the *Ling zhi*, its taste is described as bitter and the fungus was non-poisonous.

"The allusion to cinnabar is a code. Cinnabar is the blood red ore the alchemists of Europe and of the Orient obtained mercury from in efforts to prepare the mineral elixir of life. This name applied to a fungus indicates a place of the highest regard among the elixir plants. In the oldest medical text in China, *The Four Canons of Shen-nung* (B.C. 2838), cinnabar is given first among the `superior' quality medicines for attaining immortality, by which is meant superior substances for preparing elixirs of long life.

"Now because of this the name `Red Pill fungus' becomes all the more significant. The *red pill* is itself an alchemical allusion to the famous `Pill of Immortality' — the medicine made from what you in the West have called the Philosopher's stone.

"Now, while it is true such an elixir would impart *qi*, the term can also mean the `activity' of a medicine, curative force, or the `active essence.' This is equally significant to understanding the nature of the Red chi or `Ch'i fungus' of the secretive Taoists."

I was beginning to see why the old people of the Orient held this mushroom in such high esteem. Still, I wanted to learn more about it. I had to keep Dr. Wu talking. "How is it that the Ch'i fungus is now called *Ling zhi*?" I inquired.

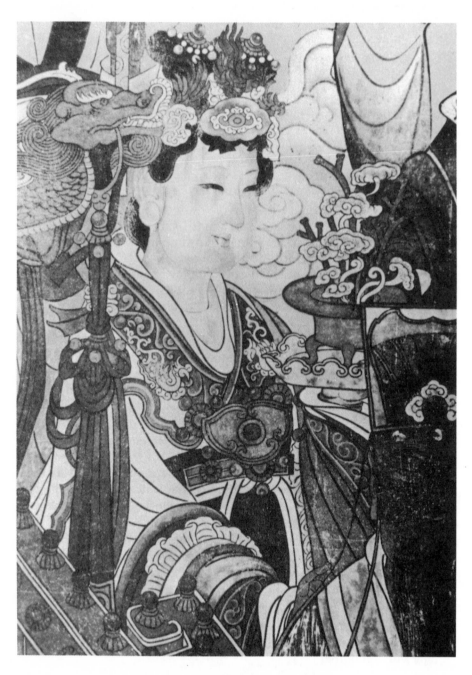

Maid of Honor, attendant to the Chinese Emperor,
carrying a vase with *Ling zhi,* including the antler form.
Painted circa 1300 A.D. (repro: Hadeler)

Dr. Wu explained, "The term *ling* doesn't appear with *chih*, or as we spell it today, *zhi*, until the 11th century when paintings of the fungus would provide mycologists in this century evidence to determine the botanical identity as *Ganoderma lucidum*. It seems it was around this time the common people learned the mushroom was highly esteemed by the shamans. Then *Ling zhi* became `shaman's fungus' or `divine chih,' *chi* or *zhi* meaning animals, plants or minerals used to concoct elixirs of long life. Therefore, Dr. Willard, *Ling zhi* could also be translated as `shaman's active ingredient.' Meanings are found within meanings."

"So someone must have gone off into the mountains where the alchemists lived and found them using it or learned its identity as the `Ch'i fungus,'" I commented.

"Yes indeed," Dr. Wu concurred. "This must have been what happened."

"But what did Li Shih-chen have to say about its medicinal use?" I wondered out loud.

Dr. Wu recalled the Taoist classics referring to the *Chi zhi* as a fungus prescribed to patients with a tight or "knotted chest." It was bitter tasting, non-poisonous and without side-effects. *Chi zhi* was said to positively affect the heart *qi*, mend the chest, cure forgetfulness and strengthen the intellect. Taken over many years it was believed to keep the body agile and allow one to live as long a life as the very immortals.

"We also see that it was possibly cultivated with the aid of special stones and plants," he recounted. "Even the cultivated mushrooms gave long life but not immortality. How the Taoists accomplished this, like many other feats of the alchemist, is unknown.

"The cultivation of this mushroom was an event that often made it into the imperial records. One famous historical incident occurred in B.C. 109 in the summer at Kan-chuan palace in one of the inner chambers (a room of ceremonial retreat). A fungus, with nine stalks, sprang up in the inner chamber of the harem. The emperor was so pleased that in a fit of generosity he ordered the distribution of wine and oxen to the people.

"This mushroom in the sleeping room of pleasure is auspicious. Many Taoists practised a special sexual art called *fang chung*, that was also thought to bring about longevity and even produce `immortality.'"

"How does this relate to the modern uses of *Fu Zheng* therapy? How would it effect AIDS and Chronic Fatigue Syndrome?" I asked.

"I think that before I answer that, I would have to give you my view of these problems," Dr. Wu said.

By this point we had recessed to a comfortable lounge. We had decided to try a fine cognac, a perfect end to a most superb meal.

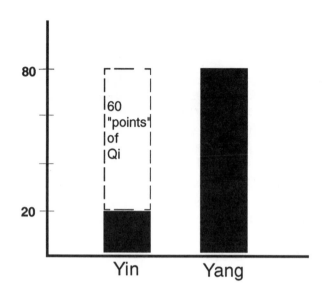

Dr. Wu's first diagram - the healthy individual

"Most AIDS victims are already essentially dead by the nature of their lifestyles," Dr. Wu began.

I didn't quite understand. "What do you mean they are already essentially dead?"

"Well, in Chinese Taoist philosophy, a homosexual is basically dead. He has cancelled out his *Qi*," Dr. Wu replied.

This statement hit me like a thunderbolt. Soldiers resurrected with a mushroom medicine was one thing — a complete condemnation of homosexuality something else entirely. I grew up during an era when Gay Rights were as important as Women's Rights, as anyone's rights. Rather horrified, I told him this was an extremely bigoted statement. Could he support it? Dr. Wu certainly liked to shock people.

"I'll draw a little graph and that will help you understand what I mean. I'm not a bit bigoted about homosexuality. As you say, it is their right, but if they don't listen to the basic, though subtle, laws of the universe, they leave themselves vulnerable to these diseases."

Taking a napkin he drew a simple graph.

"As you know, the Universe is made up of positively charged energy or *yang* energy, and negatively charged energy or *yin* energy. In

18

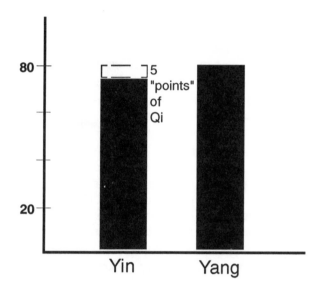

Dr. Wu's second diagram - the individual out of balance

this very simple diagram we see that the average male is of course made up of yin and yang energies. But in the gender area a male will have more yang than yin. Let's say 80 points of yang and 20 points of yin. The difference between these forces is kind of like the charge of the person.

"This is similar to being hooked up to both - and + terminals on a battery. You need both sides hooked up to have current flowing. It is the difference between the two poles that gives the charge. In our case we have a male with 60 points (80 - 20 = 60) of energy qi. The extra yang gives the male physical attributes amplified by the male genes.

"Now let us take a homosexual that has taken on a certain amount of female or yin sexuality. In this case we increase the yin to, let us say, 75 points. That means the difference between the poles is only 5 points. The energization of qi here is a very low level of 5 points. This is barely enough energy left to keep basic functions going. It is certainly not enough energy to enhance the protective energies of the immune system.

"In this devitalized state, the body is susceptible to a large range of opportunistic organisms. HIV (Human Immunodeficiency Virus) just happens to be a prominent one. It attacks the T-lymphocyte system. We would call this the yang or male part of the immune system. Since this is what is weak this is what HIV attacks.

"So I don't really feel that HIV is the cause of AIDS. I just feel it is an opportunistic virus that is feasting on a de-energized system, much as a vulture would."

"Whoa! ... that's pretty heady stuff Dr. Wu", I exclaimed. "So HIV, in your opinion, is just a scavenger cleaning up a mess. What about all the females with AIDS, the African population, etc."

"If you exclude the Africans for a moment, we still see that over 80% of the AIDS victims are male: either homosexual, hemophiliacs, or intravenous drug users. Obviously the virus can sneak past the body's defenses by direct blood transmission.

"Many of these people don't have the greatest self respect in the first place. Even most of the females are intravenous drug users and prostitutes. Again, these peoples' lifestyle is devitalizing. This is also true of many of the famine stricken people in Africa. The HIV virus has gained momentum and strength by being so widespread. But it is just doing its job, keeping a balance of energy amongst living things.

"Even the poor babies born with HIV infection have not had strong immune systems in place to resist the virus.

"Let's say we have a stagnant pool of water. In there you will find all kinds of organisms thriving, algae, insects, maybe the young of frogs, all of which are creating and living off of each other's wastes. A prominent organism, from our point of view, will also be there: the mosquito. Eighty percent of its life cycle is spent as a garbage collector in the stagnant water. The other 20% is spent in the adult stage of life biting us. Now we wouldn't say that a mosquito caused the stagnant water would we?

"The HIV story has but little difference. HIV did not cause the stagnant energy in the body. It adapts to an opening in the system, a niche. It enters in and sets up home. It holds onto that niche strongly, further paralysing the system. This of course kills the person unless further energization of the system is accomplished."

"So you're saying that all one does is re-energize the system and an AIDS person will be well again?" I said.

"In essence, yes, but of course it is never quite that easy," Dr. Wu commented.

"You see, it is a multi-level problem that is life-threatening. Once the HIV is in the body one can't just ask it to leave. It won't do that. The first significant challenge is to either stop the HIV from transforming into full AIDS or to place the AIDS into remission. Let's remember HIV doesn't kill people. It just further weakens the system so other opportunistic organisms can invade, get a foothold and further devitalize the system. It also weakens the body enough that some of the person's own fears, thoughts and genetic problems come up.

"An HIV infection, which starts to cripple the T-lymphocyte section of the immune system, is much like placing the police force out of commission. Any kind of storm or even minor disaster will send the people on a looting spree. The first stage is to declare martial law. Once we have a state of at least semi-order, then we start to revitalize the system.

"Of course this isn't always as easy as it sounds. I would have to say that the major stumbling block at this time is the patient's emotions and fears. This is often true of cancer. You can just watch the vitality recede in the average person, as soon as they hear they have the disease. The emotions and fears devitalize the body even more, letting the cancer or HIV get an even better grip on the body.

"In the case of HIV patients, these people need a spark, a reason to fight, a new joy of life. After all, the place the HIV is attacking is the military or masculine aspect of our body. These people need to vibrate strongly at that level. They need to cultivate those feelings and attitudes.

"Now that is a pretty hard thing to do when you are in a hospital bed hooked up to an intravenous tube perhaps with tubes in the nose as well. The first stage is to put out as many fires as possible. Let all the other organisms know that they are not welcome. If you can get the person back on his feet, you can then start to revitalize the system to keep the HIV in check."

"You mean to say you feel that you can keep the HIV in check so it doesn't wreak havoc in the body," I said.

"Well," he replied, "you always have a certain part of society who are criminals. You can keep the criminal elements in a society from destroying the society if you have a strong enough police force. Isolate the bad ones and you can keep the society functioning. In this case, however, I want to emphasize the emotional aspect.

"You need constant vigilance to make sure that physical structure is as vital as possible, putting out fires whenever you see them on the physical level. But if the emotions get out of hand, disease will spread like wild fire. If I have a few servants and I keep them in check, no problem. If they fan up an emotional opinion in the rest of society, you have a revolution. This is a death of the old system. This can be useful in a society that will evolve into another type of society, but in the physical body it could mean death."

"How do you see *Ling zhi* working on this?" I asked.

"*Ling zhi* will calm the body down, while revitalizing it at the same time. I'm not suggesting the *Ling zhi* is a `magic bullet' to cure AIDS, but I am saying it is an important element."

"What about Chronic Epstein-Barr virus or Chronic Fatigue Syndrome as it is now called?" I asked.

21

"I'm not that familiar with this problem. Please describe the symptoms and the nature of the patients," Dr. Wu said.

"Approximately eighty percent of the people with this problem are female," I said. "They are usually successful business women, lawyers, flight attendants, executive secretaries, school principals and so on. Most of my patients have been very healthy for years before this ailment hit them. They usually take part in some regular form of aerobic exercise program.

"Yes, I would say the largest patient category is successful, busy, business women. In North America, it has been called "Yuppie Flu" in the press. I do have a few male patients but mostly female. The syndrome is notable firstly by the general fatigue of the patients. The cause is unknown but it looks like it is caused by the Epstein-Barr virus attacking the B-lymphocyte system.

"The major symptom, as I say, is just complete fatigue. It is related to mononucleosis, with similar symptoms: sore throat, devitalized body, basically bedridden. I know of some patients that have been mostly bedridden for over a year. Going to a movie means two days of rest. It could easily be called 'burned out' syndrome. Many of these people work too hard at business and then go out to do aerobic exercise for a half hour a day. It is spreading quite fast in North America, hitting some of the most productive people in our society."

Dr. Wu said, "It almost sounds like a mirror image of the HIV story. Instead of males taking on a female role, we have females taking on a male role and thus cancelling out their own vital *qi*. I had thought that something like this would be happening."

"What do you mean?" I said.

"For every yang there has to be an equal yin to balance out the whole system. Since the T side of the lymphocyte system is being devastated mostly in males, it only makes sense that the B side of the system would be under attack in female bodies," Dr. Wu said.

"So you are again saying that this is a lifestyle problem, are you not?" I said.

"Yes."

"That is going to be a hard pill to swallow for most of my patients. I mean, I can't tell a gay male he has to start liking women instead of men and I can't tell these busy women they have to stay at home taking care of kids. They would just as soon take me out and shoot me," I replied incredulously.

Dr. Wu laughed.

"You don't have to go that far. I don't feel the right therapy here is for the physician to get shot! When a person knows they have a weakness they have to take cautionary measures to protect themselves. You would not have a person with a broken foot walk on it immediately, would you?

"Let us take the homosexual male. He does not have to stop liking males. He should probably not have any lover for a long time of course, but when he does, it should be only one, and of course only protected sex is acceptable. The most important aspect is getting in tune with his male energy. Either increase his yang energy and / or decrease his yin energy to create a bigger spark of *qi* energy.

"The same is true of the Chronic Fatigue person. They have to become more in tune with their own internal energies — stimulate some of the energy that comes with the body. A woman can still be very much a woman and be in the workplace. In China, most adult women work and have a very busy life, with poor nutrition, and still don't get this problem.

"Of course, the *Fu Zheng* herbs such as *Ling zhi*, *Huang qi*, *Gan Cao* and *Ligustrum* should be used. In the case of the female I would say no aerobic or competitive exercise and in the case of the male I would say lots of exercise which builds the body's size, and competitive exercise, of course. And as I said before, keep a constant watch to put out the fires associated with the weakened immune system until it can work by itself."

By this time we were a little tired and so we decided to part ways. Later that night as I organized my thoughts I wondered how much of Dr. Wu's comments were fantasy or myth and how much had any basis in reality. I wanted to read more about this mushroom to see if these stories had any validity.

Over the next few days, even though I had a very busy schedule, my mind kept returning to my conversation with Dr. Wu. I still wondered what parts of his tale were true. Was he just leading me on? He was considered by many to be quite reputable. I could easily confirm the story about the First Emperor of China, since the Orient abounded with these kinds of stories. I had accepted these stories as more myth than historical fact long ago. In fact, I had to say that these stories of alchemy rather excited my sense of adventure.

The problem area was really the controversy over AIDS and Chronic Fatigue Syndrome. His comments were not socially acceptable on this side of the Pacific. Dr. Wu made some very good points, as well as a new, almost refreshing look at these health problems. At first glance his ideas looked like a bigoted, moralistic, "old fashioned" point of view, based on a patriarchal regime.

A closer look gave me a new system of observing these problems, one that actually gave new hope to people who were afflicted with these diseases. Could lifestyle really affect the immune system? The obvious answer seemed to be yes! The problem is the traditional point of view of how a man and a woman should act — the yin and yang of social interaction.

It was interesting, but something that I could not likely implement at a clinical level. I didn't feel it was my place, or even appropriate, to tell a successful female business executive that to get her life in order she might have to adopt more traditional behaviour before she could be healthy.

Were there grains of truth to this, and if so how much? I couldn't quite believe that if a person were dying of AIDS, they could just change their attitude towards their sexuality and the viral infection would go into remission. I had to store this information in the category of "interesting but not substantiated."

Even if the answers were left up in the air, Dr. Wu certainly knew how to stir up some interesting questions.*

*For further reading on the ancient history of Ling zhi please consult the Notes section at the end of the book.

Chapter 2

Reishi in the Wild

Trip Home

I had spent some six weeks in the Orient, with many adventures, meeting a tremendous number of contacts. While on the long 15 hour flight to Canada my mind kept returning to Dr. Wu and our discussion on the elixir of immortality.

Of course this can't be true, I thought, it was just a story — wasn't it? Could there be a grain of truth to the stories of Reishi's ability to revitalize the body? Could this mushroom be an herb that I could use with my patients suffering from fatigue and immune deficiency? I decided that as soon as I got back I would look into it, do some research, find out if I could use it. But acquiring some *Ling zhi* to use might be almost impossible. And if the prices in Hong Kong were any indication, I wouldn't be buying very much of it.

As always after a long trip, the floodgates open wide. I was buried in work at my clinics and immediately forgot about elixirs of longevity, Reishi and Dr. Wu. Just trying to deal with daily life and the demands placed on me after my hiatus kept all of my waking hours filled.

A few months later, after seeing patients in the Vancouver clinic, I decided to visit a good friend, marketing agent Illana Holloway. Illana had moved to British Columbia's Sunshine Coast, a stretch of beautiful coastline about an hour north of Vancouver. Separated by water, the area is only accessible by combination of road and car-ferry.

As I got on the ferry I thought the name "Sunshine Coast" was rather bizarre as the coast around Vancouver was notorious for rain. It was my first time up there and I was suitably surprised. Even though it was a short 40 minute ferry ride from an overcast, cold and rainy Vancouver, it was warm and sunny up on the Sunshine Coast. Sechelt was my destination. It was almost an island, surrounded by water with only a mile wide piece of land attaching it to the mainland.

After many days cooped up in the cubicles found only in a clinic setting, I was quite happy the next day to be able to stretch my legs, fill my lungs with fresh sea air and go for a hike in some remote area along the coast. Who knows what I would find? It had been many long years since I had spent a winter in a tipi in the foothills of the Rockies. The responsibilities of teaching and work had cut back my chances to spend time in the outdoors.

As I was walking through a stretch of forest I almost fell over someone digging bracket mushrooms out of a rotting log -- the ruins of a huge alder tree.

To put it mildly, I was interested in what he was doing. Why was he harvesting the seemingly inert growth? The fellow was somewhat shaggy haired, an obvious "back-to-the-lander."

You can imagine the image that sprung to mind. The West Coast was a famous picking ground for "vision inducing" mushrooms. The mushrooms have been used by shamans throughout time and had become very popular during the '60s and '70s. But these dry, tough items didn't look like psychedelic mushrooms.

These were bracket mushrooms, shell-like growths which were saprophytic (living on dead organic matter) on hardwood logs and stumps. I remembered a time when I tried to eat a bracket mushroom back in my tipi days. I became very ill. I was poisoned by it. Though it didn't kill me, for three days I felt like it was going to. So my mind was saying that it was poisonous.

I said hello to the fellow and explained that I was an herbalist. The polyporus mushroom he had might be poisonous, I pointed out, so he'd better be careful.

He looked up at me and said he was a mycologist and that I needn't worry about him. I felt sheepish but my interest really began to peak.

"What will you be using it for?" I asked.

He told me that the bracket mushroom was known as the "herb of spiritual potency."

I stuttered, "You mean Reishi mushrooms grow along the Sunshine Coast?"

"Yes. You've heard of Reishi?" he asked.

"Well, mostly in legends. I've seen some in the exclusive herb shops of Shanghai and Hong Kong, guarded by glass, with very large price tags attached," I exclaimed.

"Well, this is much the same mushroom," he offered.

"But it doesn't look the same," I said, disbelieving.

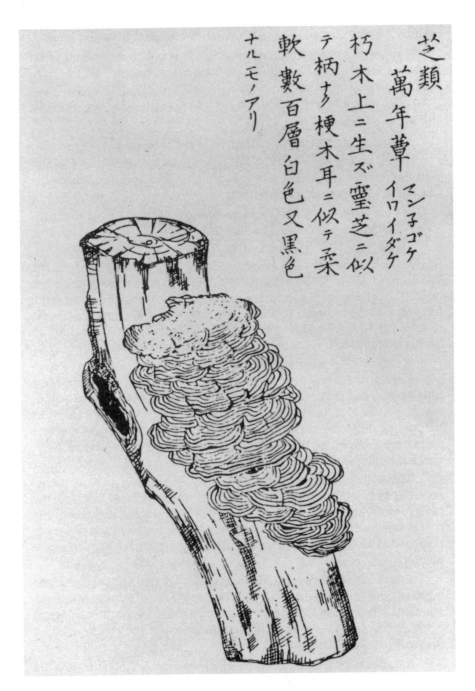

芝類
萬年蕈 マンネンゴケ イワイダケ
朽木ノ上ニ生ズ 靈芝ニ似
テ柄ヲ梗 木耳ニ似テ柔
軟 數百層 白色又黑色
ナルモノアリ

A representation of shelf mushrooms
from the Song Dynastry artist Zen -Yu Chen (repro: Hadeler)

27

"There are a few related species. This one here is *Ganoderma applanatum*, whereas the one you probably have seen is *Ganoderma lucidum*. I have it growing back at my lab if you want to have a look."

I shook my head with amazement. "This mushroom seems to be following me around the world. I can't get away from it."

The fellow introduced himself as Jeff Chilton and we started the short walk back to his lab. On the way I told him about Dr. Wu, his tales and my experience in Hong Kong.

"Who would guess it would grow here?" I blurted.

"Well, I'm a mycologist. I study mushrooms. In the process of studying fungi I realized Reishi grew on my land and throughout the coast here," Jeff politely commented.

As we walked to Jeff's lab, he recounted his relationship to mushrooms and his own history.

I could tell by Jeff's accent that he was from the U.S. As it turned out, Jeff was born and raised just across the border in Washington State. The Pacific Northwest is noted for its temperate coastal climate and high rainfall, an atmosphere conducive to a vast array of mushroom growth. Jeff grew up surrounded by evergreen forests and mushrooms underfoot. But it wasn't until he attended the University of Washington in Seattle that mushrooms became a focal point in his life.

As an undergraduate studying cultural anthropology, he became aware of the use of mushrooms for religious and medicinal purposes, a little known fact that came to light through the works of noted ethnomycologist R. Gordon Wasson. Wasson was uncovering a pattern of worldwide mushroom use that lay at the core of religious and medical prehistory. To Jeff and many others the information was fascinating. It was a turning point in his career.

The relationship between mushrooms and trees is of great economic importance to a state dependent upon forest resources, and therefore the Mycology Department at the University of Washington was one of the best in the country. Dr. Daniel Stuntz was the highly regarded professor responsible for the department and ultimately became Jeff's mycological mentor.

Courses in taxonomy and physiology broadened Jeff's understanding of mushrooms and ultimately led him to the mountains of Mexico in search of actual mushroom use by native peoples. This anthropological field trip increased his interest in mushroom use but was hampered by the real world of finances.

Returning to Seattle, broke and uncertain about the future, he visited Dr. Stuntz to relate his dilemma. The wise professor, knowing the difficulty of getting work in mycology without a Ph.D., suggested that Jeff go see Bill Street, owner of Ostrom Mushroom Farms, a local producer of button mushrooms. So Jeff went to work for Bill for the next seven years.

There was so much more to learn, and Holland was fast becoming the center for research in mushroom growing technology. Jeff applied to Holland's International Agricultural Centre and received a fellowship for three months of independent study at the Dutch School for Mushroom Growers, under the watchful eye of Pieter Vedder. The Dutch experience provided Jeff with the latest information and cultivation techniques and broadened his knowledge base.

Upon returning to Ostroms, which had just completed another expansion, he was promoted to Production Manager, responsible for the cultivation of over two million pounds of mushrooms per year.

Bill Street was not the kind of man to sit still. He had the vision to see the coming trend of exotic mushrooms that were cultivated in the Orient. He hired as his Director of Research Dr. Takahashi Urayama, a brilliant and practical Japanese mycologist who was interested in seeing Shiitake and other species produced in the U.S. Dr. Urayama brought with him strains of mushrooms and was given the mandate to start production at Ostroms. Soon, Shiitake (*Lentinus edodes*), Enokitake (*Flammulina velutipes*), and Oyster (*Pleurotus ostreatus*) mushrooms were being produced on a small commercial scale, a learning opportunity for Jeff that was to change his focus and ultimately lead to his decision to leave Ostroms in 1980 in order to concentrate on the research and cultivation of these exotic species, many of which were in fact medicinal.

During the next three years, supported by consulting work, Jeff conducted in depth research and small scale cultivation trials which resulted in *The Mushroom Cultivator: A Practical Guide to Growing Mushrooms at Home*, the most popular and widely read book on small scale mushroom cultivation yet published in the English language. This book has sold 25,000 copies and is used by some universities as a textbook. And I, of course, had the gall to suggest to Jeff on that fine sunny day that he might be poisoning himself — a man who had written a book on mushrooms!

Soon after publication of the book in 1983, Jeff emigrated to British Columbia's Sunshine Coast, an area still untouched by the population growth and the California-style development taking place in his native Washington. It was there that he built his mushroom spawn laboratory and began producing mushroom spawn for the emerging exotic mushroom industry. But having attended the Symposia on Mushroom Science in Bordeaux in 1979 and Hungary in 1986, he was convinced that the true benefits of mushrooms would come from their medicinal properties, an area finally gaining intense scientific scrutiny.

Very few mushroom growers could see this opportunity. In 1986 Jeff set up a corporation that would act as the "grow-out" facility for the medicinal mushrooms he was working with in the lab. This corporation, North American Reishi Ltd., is the first of its kind in Canada and one of but a few in North America.

Jeff's excitement about the medicinal mushroom projects as well as local harvest of the pine mushroom for export to Japan has created a new awareness of mushrooms in this small coastal community.

We emerged from the woods into a large clearing. At the top of the clearing was a modern cedar log home, one of the kind commonly built as summer homes before the price of cedar went so high. Fifty feet away was a 1000 sq. ft. building that could only be the lab, the blue green metal siding providing sharp contrast to the warm cedar home. We entered the front door into a clean white office. His bookshelves were full of more mushroom books than I'd seen in any bookstore and dried mushroom specimens were filling another set of shelves.

He pointed to his Macintosh computer and noted that it was the central focus for information gathering and experiment tracking, without which he would be swamped in a sea of unmanageable data. As a fellow computer enthusiast I could only nod in agreement.

Before we could go through the door into the next room, we had to remove our shoes and outer garments. Jeff explained that our walk through the woods had most certainly covered us with spores of many micro-organisms — contaminants in lab terms. The adjacent room was long and narrow, with a large metal door at one end. Dials and control knobs were arrayed above it. This was the autoclave where all his spawn growing media was sterilized, he explained, opening the heavy stainless steel door revealing a deep inner chamber.

Standing next to it was a smaller autoclave which was used for preparing agar media and sterilizing culture tools. A steam boiler and stainless steel culture tanks were in the room behind the autoclaves. This high tech facility was a maze of doors, necessary to maintain the sterility of the inner culture areas.

"In fact," he said, "I can only let you stand in the doorway and look into the inoculation room."

This room with its white walls and white metal shelves would have made any scientist proud.

"What, pray tell, are those?" I said, pointing to the large boxes with shiny corrugated surfaces.

"Those are my laminar flow hoods," he replied. "The corrugated surface is the face of a high efficiency particulate filter, through which a fan blows air. The filter scrubs the air in this room of any spores, bacteria, or dust particles. I do all my work in front of those filters, which effectively provide me with a sterile working space."

"Oh," I said, trying to look as though I'd caught everything he had said.

"All it takes is one microscopic spore to spoil my work. So you can see why this room has to be so clean."

We moved on to the next room which was for incubation. Racks with gallon jars of cooked grain filled the room. The grain was covered with what looked like white mold.

"I see you're pretty good at growing molds," I said.

Smiling, Jeff replied, "In fact, that white mold you see is actually the mushroom organism that I'm growing. It's called mycelium and is the true body of the fungus organism. It colonizes the grain, which then becomes a seed to a mushroom grower, who mixes the mycelium-covered grain into his substrate, whether it be compost or straw or wood of some sort.

"This is pure-culture grain spawn and is due to be shipped out to an Oyster mushroom grower this week.

"But you might be more interested in this," he said pointing to some plastic bags on shelves. My jaw fell open when I saw Reishi (the one I was used to seeing on glass counters in stores). Nearby were Shiitake mushrooms growing in trays — the same Shiitake that was my regular fare in sushi bars. Then I saw the special one.

The base of the plastic bag contained a 5 inch deep dense growth of whitish mycelium with some yellow overtones. But growing on the surface of the white growth in the humid chamber above it were long reddish antler shapes, creamy white at the tips.

"Reishi," I proclaimed, "the rare antler form!"

"Very astute," said Jeff, "*Ganoderma lucidum* it is. And allow me to let you in on a little secret. The antler form can be caused simply by raising the carbon dioxide level of the air in the chamber, a phenomenon common to many mushroom species. Similarly, light or the absence of it can affect the amount of pigment a mushroom produces and hence its color can vary. But in nature the antlered form was undoubtedly the rarest of them all. This no doubt made it quite special.

"There has been a tremendous amount of research on *Ganoderma* in the last few years, especially by the Japanese," Jeff commented.

"How does it shape up compared to the Shiitake mushroom?" I asked.

"I feel that Reishi is clearly more potent, especially the newly developed Chinese strains I'm working with," Jeff replied.

"Reishi's high polysaccharide content is thought to be responsible for its immune stimulating effect. In fact, Reishi is presently being used in San Francisco clinics treating the AIDS community, who feel they are getting reasonable results. It has also been used on Chronic Fatigue Syndrome sufferers (CFS)."

31

I was dumbfounded. I was reflecting on my plane ride and the words of Dr. Wu. I didn't say a word to Jeff. I just wanted to listen.

Jeff continued," Traditionally, Reishi has been used for what is called 'aging blood,' specifically for arteriosclerosis, heart problems, high blood pressure, blood clots, insomnia, nervous conditions, toxic liver and stomach problems. It is specifically useful for allergic asthma."

"Can anyone just go out and pick it? I mean, is it easy to find?" I asked in disbelief.

"The problem with amateurs going Reishi-hunting is that the fungus looks similar to some poisonous mushrooms, and that could lead to serious problems!" Jeff exclaimed.

"Is the information you're outlining about the medicinal quality of Reishi solid? Have there been clinical studies and lab tests or is it mostly folklore?" I asked.

We walked over to a filing cabinet and he pulled out a rather large file. "There are about 15 studies here but I'm sure you could find a lot more if you looked hard," Jeff replied.

A brief glance and I saw amazing titles: *Studies on Fungal Polysaccharides, Anticancer and Immunostimulant Polysaccharides, Fu Zheng Herbs in the Treatment of Cancer, Clinical Observations on Hypoglycemia Treatment with Ling zhi (Ganoderma) tablets.*

The research looked pretty good. "Can I get some copies of these papers?" I inquired.

"Sure, I'll photocopy them and send them off to you next week."

Jeff gave me a small antlered Reishi to take with me and promised to show me the North American Reishi grow-out facility on my next visit. I gave Jeff my address and left his lab in a bit of a daze.

Here was Reishi again! I had thought this was an intriguing Oriental mystery and here was the mushroom growing wild and cultivated little more than an hour from my own clinic.

There was little doubt that the time was overdue for a serious investigation of the literature on Reishi.

When I got back to my friend Illana's place, I relayed the whole story to her. She laughed and noted that I certainly didn't live a boring life. We both got excited about the events of the weekend. I asked her if she could do a little checking around and find out more about Jeff, his lab and his interest in mushrooms.

The next day I was back on a plane to Calgary. I couldn't wait to sit down at my computer. Over the years I had many occasions to do research on plant-medicines. Like many researchers around the world today, I take advantage of the massive scientific databases which are available "on-line." Sitting at home, I dial up a phone number with my computer's modem (a special attachment). Using special codes and passwords, I gain access to the DIALOG system, a central database from which I could search many others.

Returning home I immediately went to the computer to dial up DIALOG, typed in "file 5 - Biosis -" thinking it would be the best bet. Sure enough, when I entered the key words GANODERMA and REISHI, the computer responded with a series of "hits." The "hits" indicated that there were scientific papers relating to those topics somewhere in the database.

Another amazing aspect of modern technology. The phone line buzzes, a computer in Palo Alto, California reacts to my request and in a matter of seconds searches millions of scientific papers, flashing back on my screen that 220 papers had been written with those key words since 1969.

Bingo! I had uncovered a hotbed of research. Don't get excited, I told myself, these papers might be on Reishi as an insecticide or food colouring — something way off the point. A quick look through the titles of the articles, however, reassured me that most of them were solid pieces of research on the health effects of the plant. I "downloaded" the abstracts and in less than five minutes I had created enough reading material on this mushroom to last me many months. I could be pretty confident that this list included at least 75% of the papers written on the subject since 1969.

It made for amazing reading. Reishi was obviously a significant focus of research for pharmaceutical labs during the previous fifteen years. I felt reassured about Reishi's reputation in myth. Often when I search the literature by computer, only one or two papers will appear. Here I had well over two hundred pieces of scientific research, all on the same plant that Dr. Wu had so eloquently praised.

After collecting my computer information, I immediately went to my own research library. Over the years I've collected hundreds of books and photocopies on herbal medicine. My Chinese section was hardly "world-class," but it had been growing rapidly in the past few years. My first stop was the Oriental herbals — the giant volumes which summarize the range of herbs, minerals and animal products used in Oriental medicine. The results were rather disappointing. Then I found a reference to Reishi in a major book.

The minutes passed with no more luck. My choices were fewer and fewer. It looked as though my own library of Chinese books would be little help. I needed a new tack. I spread my search wider to encompass general references on Oriental history and texts on the history of herbal medicine around the world. I checked books of myth, tomes on alchemy and the history of society, category after category. In each area I would find a page or two, perhaps only a paragraph. Slowly but surely, I built up my stack of reference works. In an hour there were 21 books and articles in a pile on my library floor.

When I added my pile to the materials Jeff Chilton had sent, I had a fistful of information on this herb — both from science and folklore.

I phoned Illana to share my excitement, telling her that I had good news and bad news. The good news was that I had found lots of scientific papers to substantiate some of the claims about Reishi. The bad news was that I would need an elixir of longevity myself just to go through all the material. My schedule was already overburdened but I felt this information really needed to get out to the general public.

"It sounds on the surface like it's just the herb we need in North America at this time," she said.

She assured me, as she always does, that "something will break through. A way will show itself and the information will reach the people who need it."

Chapter 3

Reishi in Medical Science

The next week Illana phoned and said, "Guess what. A friend of mine was in the local newspaper office the other day with one of your books and a guy comes up to her and asked if she knew you. She said no, but that she had a friend who did, and the long and short of it is he phoned me. He knows Jeff and said he talked to you on a few occasions a couple years ago. His name is Ken Jones, and he does literature searches on natural products and lives just five miles up the coast."

"Ken Jones," I thought, searching back through dozens of researchers and herbalists that I had met through the years. "Oh yes, about two years ago I was doing a research project on Lapacho (or Pau D'Arco). Ken was also doing some research on the plant and once I met him in person."

"Would you like to meet him to see if he can help you on the Reishi research? He's right here on the coast, has seen Jeff's operation and has already gathered a fair amount of material on the subject. He might be able to help you wade through some of the papers on Reishi."

It sounded good to me so the following week, after I finished at the Vancouver clinic, I took another Sunday ferry up to Sechelt. I met Ken at Illana's place overlooking Porpoise Bay on Sechelt Inlet. The nearby airport navigation light steered seaplanes to the dock on the bay. Her place was a pleasant condo townhouse filled with miniature statues and Van Gogh prints. Its open beam construction and large windows made it very homey. The view out the windows was virtually a wilderness setting.

Within minutes of meeting, Ken and I were talking about all kinds of issues surrounding natural pharmaceuticals. It didn't take long to get around to the dynamic research on polysaccharides, substances that had been found in many plants. Some of these molecules had immune-modulating characteristics, affecting the overall defense mechanisms of animals and humans.

Before I knew it a few hours had gone by. Illana came back in with some tea. She laughed and warned us that our conversation was deadly boring to anyone who wasn't a biochemist. No surprise to me. I had seen the glaze appear over more than one set of eyes when I began talking about the physiological effects of herbs!

We went out onto Illana's open patio and had a little snack with our tea. I found that Ken was a very intelligent man, with a great background in medicinal plant research and a solid understanding of natural medicine. A rare find to say the least. We decided we could work together on the Reishi project.

We wanted to get the information both in encapsulated form and with full detail if the area seemed to be of importance. I thought to myself, "Let's see how many of these myths are true."

The first area of interest for me was the topic of immune modulation. The Chinese refer to it as *Fu Zheng* therapy. So Ken Jones and I left our first meeting with plenty to do — he with a stack of papers and ideas, myself with a growing list of questions.

Fu Zheng

I was first introduced to *Fu Zheng* by Dr. Paul Lee, a noted herbal researcher who lives rather idyllically on the coast of California in the small city of Santa Cruz. With a name like Lee and a subject matter like *Fu Zheng*, you might think Dr. Lee is Chinese, but that couldn't be farther from the truth.

Dr. Lee is the quintessential North American scholar. A burly man topping out at over 6 feet; with his neatly trimmed grey beard and effusive manner, no one would mistake him for Oriental. He seems more like one of the majestic redwoods which grow not too far from where he lives. Educated at Harvard with a doctorate in theology, he worked as a teaching assistant to the famous philosopher, Paul Tillich. Dr. Lee's knowledge of the roots of Western culture is awe inspiring. His formal education is matched by many years of industrious research on herbs, medical history and medical philosophy.

Dr. Lee was the leader of the People to People delegation which was my first introduction to mainland China. The group was focusing on Chinese herbal medicine and the herbal manufacturing industry. Every place we went on that six week trip, people expected Paul to be Chinese. The number of Li's (pronounced Lee) or Lee's in China would probably fill a nation in other parts of the world.

Paul's knowledge extended to Oriental medical traditions and one which he mentioned to me was *Fu Zheng*.

He told me, "I was first introduced to *Fu Zheng* by Dr. Sun Yan, head of cancer surgery at the Beijing Cancer Hospital. He was visiting the

University of Texas in Houston where he was asked to do three or four years of research on herbs that could stop the side-effects of both chemotherapy and radiation therapy associated with cancer.

"To do this he reinstated the ancient concept of *Fu Zheng* therapy. This is similar to Brekhman's work in the USSR on adaptogen uses of Siberian ginseng and that of Wagner in Germany on *Echinacea* at the University of Munich in the therapy called *umstimmungstherapie*, which translates literally as `to retune.'

"These three scholars seem to be the most important in Europe, the USSR and China in this area of research. Sun Yang's work on *Fu Zheng* was mostly with *Ligustrum* and *Astragalus*."

Fu Zheng is really the correlate to Western immunotherapy. *Fu Zheng* plants (one of which is Reishi) are employed to increase disease-resistance and normalize body functions. Specifically, substances are used to treat deficient principles of *qi*, the "vital" or life energy, blood, and yin (fluid) and yang function (especially kidney).

These are not the ordinary categories that Westerners expect to work with. Nonetheless, each of these terms means something concrete to the traditional Oriental medical physician. Reishi has a place of importance as a *qi*-tonic along with the herbs *Astragalus* and ginseng. *Qi* may be best defined as "life energy." Different than electricity yet mimicking its ability to "flow," *qi* (or *ch'i* as it is sometimes spelled) supports and nourishes life in all living things.

In modern times, *Fu Zheng* herbs are given the added task of decreasing the side-effects of Western medical procedures (such as surgery, radio- and chemotherapies), which can sometimes weaken a patient's immune system. Traditionally, *Fu Zheng* herbs were also used to moderate the activities of herbs which were used to destroy cancerous and other abnormal cells.

Modern diagnostic techniques have allowed the physicians of the Orient to combine Western and Eastern medical techniques — a process which nonetheless requires a great deal of monitoring.

When my delegation went to Beijing, we spent a whole day exchanging papers on this subject at the Beijing Science Hall. Dr. Sun Yan was there as was Dr. Wang Tun, Director of Training at the Chinese Pharmaceutical Corporation. Other dignitaries included Dr. Lou Zhicen, Professor of Pharmacognosy and President of the Chinese Pharmaceutical Association, Dr. Cao Chunling, Director of the Department of Chinese Pharmacy at Beijing College of Traditional Chinese Medicine and Dr. Sun Nanjun, Institute of Medicinal Plant Development and Director of the Chinese Society of Traditional and Natural Drugs.

We discussed many aspects of herbal study but concentrated on the immunostimulating properties of plants. Each of our delegates and each of theirs gave a paper on related areas. We continued our discussion in both formal and informal manner over a feast of justly famous Peking duck — a type said to be found only in the city itself.

Throughout the two weeks of our trip, *Fu Zheng* was one of the most important topics. One of the major researchers in the modern development of immune-modulation in China is a woman professor, Dr. Li. My meeting with her at the Shanghai Institute of Materia Medica during the People to People visit had stimulated me sufficiently to revisit her and Dr. Xu Rensheng. During the group visit we discussed immune modulating plants and the concept of *Fu Zheng* for some three hours, but it wasn't until a visit some four months later that Dr. Li and I discussed Reishi in any depth.

Back to Canada

After that first trip to the mainland I returned to Canada with a growing of interest in Oriental herbs. I was getting to the point where I could ask intelligent questions when I ran into experts on the topic. What had Ken Jones found out in the intervening weeks? On my next trip to the Vancouver clinic I got in touch with him.

Ken began, "In keeping with its ancient reputation, practitioners of traditional medicine regarded Reishi as a kind of tonic that restores the "vital" or life energy, which they still refer to as *qi* or *Ch'i*."

"Where does this fit into Western physiology?" I asked.

"Well," he replied, "increasing our resistance to disease is a common theme with *Ganoderma* in traditional medicine and in the laboratory."

"*Wei Qi*," I said. "The Chinese have a special kind of *qi* called *Wei Qi* that can be compared to a military general and an army.

"*Wei Qi* is adesignated as the military *qi*, or protective energy. The normal types of *qi* flow through vessels such as blood vessels. Blood is full of *qi*. *Wei Qi* is on the outside of the vessels, protecting the vessels and the body.

"It is interesting to note that the game the Japanese call *Go*, the Chinese call *Wei Qi*. It is a military strategy game. The goal is protecting your own territory while surrounding your opponent's territory. This game was greatly revered by the same Taoists that have all of the myths about Reishi. We can say that *Wei Qi* is part of our immune function, similar to the T-lymphocytes. But *Wei Qi* is more like an electrical force than a biochemical or cellular force. The Chinese talk more about the `electrical wiring' than they do about the cells. Are these metaphors, or is it another level of reality?"

38

RNA from Reishi disrupts viral diseases by inducing interferon production.*

Ken responded, "An intriguing case in point occurred in 1979 when Polish investigators discovered a *Ganoderma* by-product of value in antiviral research.

"At the Institute of Microbiology and Biochemistry at the University of M. Curie-Sklodowska, researchers found that intravenous injections of ribonucleic acid (RNA) from the fruit body of *G. applanatum* prolonged the life of mice when given at various times before a lethal dose of a virus known as tick borne encephalitis virus."

"So RNA from Reishi delayed the occurrence of a lethal viral disease in mice. How did it do this?" I said.

Ken said, "The protective action was shown to be due to the induction of interferon."[30]

"Ah, that's really interesting." I scratched my chin a bit. Interferon is a substance the body secretes to protect itself from viral infection. Western immunologists are very interested in anything which affects interferon levels in the body. Ken explained that the reason for administering the RNA beforehand is that interferon's benefits are not geared to cells that are already infected, but as the name suggests, it interferes with the virus invading the cell, aiding those still in need of protection from the multiplication of invading viruses. "Was there any associated research on this topic?" I asked.

Ken referred to his notes. "There was some *in vitro* work done. In a culture dish, the same RNA provided normal cells with 90% protection against the *vaccinia* virus. Everyone noted that more work needed to be done on the subject.[30] The RNA is found in the fruit body of *Ganoderma lucidum* and in higher levels in the mycelium[31] — the fine thread-like structure from which the mushroom emerges."

A tantalizing possibility, I thought, but not much work on the subject. "What else?" I asked, glancing out the window and counting four blue herons standing in the bay.

"Not surprisingly," Ken began, "the scientists have been busy seeing if Reishi and its derivatives had any effects on bacteria. If it influenced the body's ability to handle viruses then it was a good bet it would do the same against bacteria."

---

* For those who would prefer to skim the scientific sections, simply read the summaries in the shaded boxes.

> ## Reishi inhibits bacteria: *Staphylococci, Streptococci* and *Bacillus pneumoniae.*

"Reishi is listed as bacteriostatic, cell-inhibiting we might say, to *staphylococci, streptococci* and *Bacillus pneumoniae* by the OHAI people (Oriental Healing Arts Institute) in their materia medica. Researchers in Taiwan tested mice with lethal doses of the bacteria *E. coli.*[32]

"They fed the mice a water extract of Reishi 48 hours before the *E. coli* injection but it had no effect. Several studies with an injection of Reishi extract 48 hours before the *E. coli* injections showed dramatic preventive ability. Anywhere from 60 - 85% of the mice survived in a situation where the control group suffered 100% fatality."[33]

> ## Polysaccharides - (long branched chains of sugar) seem to be the main immune-modulators in Reishi.

"The key element, according to the researchers seemed to be the polysaccharides — they seem to have a modulating effect on the immune system," Ken finished.

"I'll bet they're right. It isn't unusual. Many of the plants I've done research on, such as Echinacea and Chlorella, have polysaccharides as important active constituents. Do we have any specific information on Reishi polysaccharides?" I asked.

> ## Polysaccharides increase RNA and DNA in the bone marrow where immune cells such as lymphocytes are made.

"There's some promising research on one polysaccharide in particular," Ken began. He reached for a thick file folder stuffed with photocopies. "There's one simply called D6. Researchers in Beijing injected it into mice for a week and then monitored the changes in RNA and DNA in the bone marrow. Increases were roughly 50%. Protein in bone marrow also increased by as much as 28.5%.[34]

"It's in the bone marrow that the body manufactures B-cells which in turn produce antibodies. It's also where macrophages have some of their earliest beginnings. I'd say this discovery may well hold future significance in clinical applications of Reishi extractives to cancer patients. The authors of this study, commenting on the marked influence D6 exhibits on protein and nucleic acid metabolism, as well as the enhancement of protein synthesis, believe these actions provide both the basis of Reishi's traditional role as a *Fu Zheng* herb — supporting the `healthy energy' and strengthening the resistance of the body — and the `material basis of the multiple pharmacological activities attributed to this herb.'"[35]

"An intriguing start but what about specific mechanisms for polysaccharide activities extracted from *Ganoderma*?" I asked him.

Decoction of Reishi produces immune-enhancing response in mice.

"There have been certain difficulties in arriving at the exact mechanisms involved," he agreed. "Unspecific as they may yet be, the findings speak of definite immune cell activity enhancement — strengthening the resistance of the body and supporting the `healthy energy.' Investigators in China found that the polysaccharide part of Reishi, which is largely made up of amino acids and low molecular weight polysaccharides, causes a marked increase in the action of macrophages to gobble up foreign cells in the abdomen of mice.[34] And in Japan, working with *G. applanatum*, researchers at the Drug Research Institute of the Toyama Medical and Pharmaceutical University established immune enhancement in mice in response to herbal decoctions and injections.

"In some cases, double the dose provided only half the enhancement.[35] A Korean study on Reishi extract noted enhanced ability of leucocytes to go after *E. coli*, and they found lower dosages more effective than higher ones.[36]

"And here's an interesting aspect." He reached over and handed me a wad of photocopies.

Reishi augments immunoglobulin G and expands the "memory" of T-cells.

"Experiments at the Drug Research Institute in Toyama, Japan, confirmed that polysaccharides are responsible for the immune enhancement and it appears the crude extract of the Ancient *Ling zhi* (*G. applanatum*) augments the responsiveness of antibodies — particularly immunoglobulin G (IgG) — by expanding the so-called `memory' of T-cells,[35] most likely involving helper T-cells.[37] As you know, IgG constitutes a

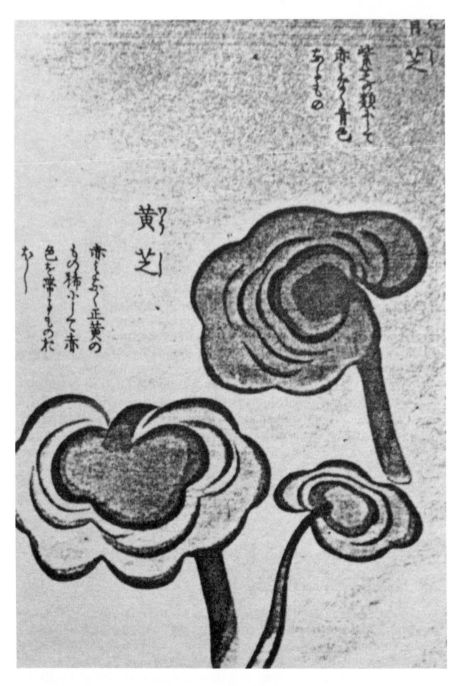

Representation of Reishi
from the Japanese book "Ben Cao Tu Pu" (repro: Hadeler)

major class of antibodies in human serum that act to enhance *phagocytosis* (the cell-gobbling action of certain immune cells) and neutralize toxins. Deficiencies are known to be associated with recurrent infections of the respiratory tract,[38] which just happens to be one of the most common applications of *Ganoderma* in traditional Chinese medicine."

I was sitting there looking at a few statues of old Chinese emperors which Illana had set on the coffee table. "So," I said, "we've got lots of mouse-based research out of the Orient. Research with extracts have definite effects on the bone marrow activity, antibody response and so on. Everyone is a bit mystified about the specific biochemistry of the effects but in general the effects match up with what the ancient Chinese doctors used Reishi for."

"That's about it," answered Ken.

"How about the areas of AIDS and CFS, Ken?" I asked. This was an area of great interest, especially after my conversation with Dr. Wu.

"It looks like there has been quite a bit of interest, at least by the non-allopathics. A newsletter out of San Francisco called *AIDS Treatment NEWS* talks about research conducted on *Fu Zheng* treatment of AIDS by Dr. Dharmananda and his group. Reishi is one of the herbs that appears to be used successfully. Shiitake is another.

"There's quite an interest, it seems, in any elixir of longevity for the immune system. Reishi is certainly getting its share. Indications are that both Reishi and Shiitake will be major participants in this arena in the future."

"*HerbalGram* has been following some of these areas also," I stated. "I'm quite interested in this area, as it has very direct and current clinical applications with many of my patients. Dr. Wu gave me some rather loose ideas about lifestyle that seem to be getting some results. I feel that some combination of lifestyle, nutrition and *Fu Zheng* type herbs and vitamins might be the answer to put at least some of these immune syndrome diseases into remission.

"I'm certainly having great success with CFS. Especially when lifestyle changes are also introduced."

Reishi is officially listed as a substance for treating cancer by the Japanese Government.

"The immune modulating effect doesn't seem to be only at the endocrine level," I continued. "There's plenty of evidence for its effective use on cancer. In fact I've heard it is an officially listed substance to be used on cancer, recognised by the Japanese government in light of recent information. As I say I've no specific reference for this but its special area of use is to overcome side-effects of Western chemotherapy and radiation therapy."

"Now that's worth reviewing right away. The Japanese labs are some of the best in the world," Ken pointed out.

Cancer

Ken reached for a pile of material and waved it in the air. "In comparison to its other properties, Reishi has received by far the most attention as a source of antitumor activity. Once again this action is due to immunostimulating `polysaccharides,' particularly those known as *Beta*-glucans. Before we look into the work that's gone on with Reishi and these complex sugars, it's important to have a perspective of the topic at hand. Some background information on the search for immunostimulants and their use in medicine will go a long way in explaining the potential of Reishi against cancer.

"Actually, Terry, I've got a great story to tell you about a Japanese physician working with Reishi.

"The Orient is no longer the only place where Reishi has a reputation as a folk-treatment for cancer. Accounts of cancer remissions attributed to the fungus are current in Canada and the U.S. too. But testimonies such as these, encouraging as they may be, are not enough to rely on for the successful treatment of any particular kind of cancer.

"Long term clinical studies with Reishi to determine which cancers will respond better than others, and by how much, have not been conducted. Without them treating cancer using Reishi alone constitutes a desperate experiment. However so, in cases considered terminal, when the patient is too weak to endure the toxicity of conventional therapies, few physicians today would argue against the attempt."

> Long-term treatment of cancer with Reishi has success.

"One such physician is Fukumi Morishige, M.D., Dr. Med. Sci., Ph.D., a former heart surgeon and now cancer surgeon who for over 30 years has routinely administered mega-doses of vitamin C to his patients, originally to facilitate better healing of their wounds following surgery. After a visit to his hospital by Dr. Linus Pauling in 1975, at Morishige's invitation, his interest eventually turned to the use of the vitamin in the treatment of cancer. A report on his studies and treatment innovations with terminal cancer patients given bone marrow transplants and a form of vitamin C known as nucleic acid ascorbate (10 grams/day), to counter the immuno-compromising effects of chemotherapy, appears in *Vitamins and Cancer: Human Cancer Prevention by Vitamins and Micronutrients.* (Humana Press, 1986).[39]

"In 1987 he delivered a talk to the Kampo I-yaku Shimbun (Herbal Medicine Press) of Tokyo, giving a pre-publication report of his clinical results with Reishi at a cancer hospital, results that so amazed him he was led to conclude that Reishi, more than perhaps any other substance he knows of, can fill the role of cancer preventive and curative. That may seem a pretty idle statement, but a full report of his clinical and experimental findings is due out soon. Let me summarize his press conference in Tokyo. It reflects the latest information on the clinical application of Reishi in Japan.

"In the spring of 1986, after 36 years wielding a scalpel, Morishige retold how he had found himself in an opportune position as counselor in a cancer hospital to explore his suspicion that there may be something inherently superior to surgery — a way to induce the body to heal itself. With an idealist's yearning for a non-invasive therapy for cancer, he began his experiments with Reishi, though at first with disappointment. Morishige explained that in low doses in various diseases the results were so unsatisfactory that for a time he believed the fungus was ineffective. But that would change forever with the arrival of a bed-ridden patient, a woman of 39 suffering from lung cancer and cancerous pleurisy, a disease complication particularly difficult to treat — so difficult in fact, that physician after physician had refused even to operate.[40]

"She had come to him as her last hope of surviving. He recounted how he examined her after six months and found an unusual absence of swelling and a much improved picture on the X-ray shots of her chest. Some swelling and only a trace amount of the cancer appeared at the lower left lung. What had she been doing? This was not the diagnostic picture presented six months ago. It turned out that all during her ordeal her husband had been out scouring the forests for Reishi and then decocting the harvest for her to drink. Morishige figured she had taken approximately a 4 gram dose per day. There being no reason to suspect further complications from exploratory surgery, he operated to see what had happened. There was no tumor left; only scars. The tissue sample he removed from the place on the X-ray that had shown a trace of cancer remaining was filled with cancerous cells, but benign ones! It was this experience that prompted him to begin administering Reishi and vitamin C in large doses. What he would discover with the forces of this fungus and the vitamin combined astounded him all the more."[40]

> Vitamin C appears to increase the absorbability of Reishi polysaccharides, improving treatment of cancer and other types of diseases.

"A large dose of Reishi, which he gives as 2 to 9 grams/day, produced diarrhea. When a large dose of vitamin C (6 to 12 grams/day) was combined however, no diarrhea occurred. Since it was already known that high molecular weight polysaccharides have this effect (which owes to their difficulty being absorbed) he figured the vitamin C could be lowering their molecular weight. Among the 240 patients he had been randomly administering Reishi and vitamin C, he also noticed that among 60 cancer patients on the combination there were notably less infections. And another curious thing happened. In those patients who had shown high readings of immunoglobulins (IgA, IgG, IgE, IgM), their counts had lowered, while those who previously had low counts now showed the same antibodies in higher counts. Could it be, he wondered, that an immunopotentiating effect of Reishi polysaccharides was being enhanced by the vitamin, making their absorbability greater? It appeared this was indeed the case.[40]

"Morishige went on to explain that his own animal studies had shown high rates of antitumor activity with the fungal polysaccharide PS-K derived from a bracket mushroom called *Kawaratake* (*Coriolus versicolor*), but that he did not find these kinds of remission rates in human cancer patients,[40] a fact that with some exceptions is apparent with the current prescription of this polysaccharide in cancer. Generally, unless the patient is terminal, PS-K is only approved for use in combination with conventional treatment approaches."[9]

"So why do animals get these phenomenally high rates of cancer remission and people don't?" I asked.

"Morishige has reason to believe the difference lies in the fact that whereas we humans must obtain our vitamin C from external sources, animals produce their own supply of the vitamin right inside their bodies. With this ability, he believes, they are capable of rendering high molecular weight polysaccharides, such as the immunostimulating ones in Reishi (mol. wt. 10,000 to 1,050,000) to a molecular weight of 30,000 when they become `oligoglucans' with 2 to 6 units of simple sugars rather than the large numbers typical of polysaccharides. They are then much more readily absorbed in the intestines and bloodstream.[40]

"His experiments so far indicate that this is indeed what is happening,[40] and would explain the remarkable remissions found in his patients.

As the cases Morishige related in 1987 portend, he may very well have discovered a revolutionary means of immunotherapy and perhaps of cancer prevention too.

"Following surgery for breast cancer, a woman of 50, deteriorating with metastasizing lung cancer, started on Reishi at a dose of approximately 6 grams a day. She continued the treatment for a period of six months, at which point she could breathe without difficulty and had no sign of the tumor remaining. Her treatment with Reishi went on, however, as a cautionary measure. Morishige included a similar case of breast cancer which invaded the bones. The patient was in extreme pain with no mobility below her head. After two months on Reishi (9 to 12 grams/day) she became free from pain, was walking, and in short was ordered discharged.[40]

"Morishige successfully treated a man diagnosed with rectal cancer which had spread to affect the liver. Dramatic improvement was evident after six months on Reishi (6 grams/day). In another case, a man of 60 with cancer of the pancreas made a complete recovery on Reishi (9 grams/day intravenously). He returned to work on a maintenance dose of 5 grams Reishi per day. Morishige added that there are not just a few cases like these, but many others, including cases of hepatitis and high blood pressure successfully treated with Reishi combined with vitamin C.[40]

"In 1979 Kosai Matsumoto II presented the first English language book on the popular use of Reishi, expounding accounts of cures 'too numerous to mention.'[3] His book, *The Mysterious Reishi Mushroom* (Woodbridge Press, Santa Barbara), though now outdated, brought Western attention to a rare fungus. Reishi had only been successfully cultivated commercially in the last 30 years, and only since the appearance of his book on any sizeable scale. Before then, scant availability and considerable expense made Reishi a treasure for the privileged few.

"Matsumoto gave examples of cancer patients consuming Reishi who lived well beyond the time they were expected to. And while some later died, other testimonies sent to him were from patients still improving, a final outcome unknown. He found these patients unanimous in claiming improved appetite, bowel movement and elimination of pain.[3] In one remarkable case, a 57-year-old man had no other treatment and was still in remission from stomach cancer five years later.[4]

"Matsumoto summarized the approach taken in modern China. In that country, ancient principles are adhered to though the active parts of extracts of polypores are incorporated. In his book,Matsumoto explains this as follows:

'The practitioners of Chinese medicine do not, of course, use polypores alone for the treatment of cancer. They administer the anticancer components of the polypores to the patient combined with various other medicines. It is different from just giving the patient an anti-cancer agent that is good only for killing cancerous cells. The method of treatment used in Chinese medicine is designed to increase appetite, restore mental powers, provide necessary elements for various bodily functions, and cure the cancer. It is a four-fold way of treating cancer that amounts to what is known these days as 'immunotherapy.'"[6]

"Did he explain what he meant by a `four-fold way?'" I inquired.

"No, but as a matter of fact," Ken offered, "we're right back to *Fu Zheng* therapy here. The four-fold approach Matsumoto referred to corresponds with a category for which *Fu Zheng* herbs are used in treating deficient principles of (1) *qi*, the "vital" or life energy, (2) blood, (3) yin (fluid) and (4) yang function (especially kidney). As you know, there are tonics for each principle, Reishi being *primarily* a *qi* tonic, along with the representative herbs *Astragalus* and ginseng."[2]

Reishi wakes up the immune system early to fight cancer, helping to prevent it.

"More research is required to learn exactly what is occurring at the cellular level. Immunologically, Morishige has no doubt that macrophages are being stimulated and to a highly significant degree. Once the oligoglucans are dissolved in the bloodstream, the macrophage, which he explains normally rests until late in the war on abnormal and foreign cells, is called into action at an earlier stage of the battle. Morishige likes to use the analogy of a lion in sleep rudely awakened by the oligoglucan produced in the system from Reishi.

"The same action might also provide an effective means of controlling cancer. Morishige estimates that the early detection of one in a hundred cases is a good rate. But he points out that even with monthly checkups, 25% will go undetected. The technology needed to improve these odds is simply not available. Because of this situation, he adds, cancer prevention must go hand in hand with early detection. And if the sleeping lion of the immune system could be awakened earlier on, prevention might be so much the better.[40]

"As studies were proceeding he couldn't say what other immune cells are involved, but that the long work ahead to answer this and other questions attending the dynamics of the treatment would proceed. To this he gave his solemn assurance."[40]

"So Dr. Morishige is putting his reputation on the line to place Reishi in the modern medical pharmacopoeia. What about other research on this general subject? Does Reishi have a history of research in Japan otherwise?" I asked.

Ken continued, "The ancient unbroken traditional belief in Japan that polypores (hardened bracket mushrooms) are useful in treating cancers[28] surfaced again in 1964 when a report had reached the U.S. National Cancer Institute that people in Japan used *G. applanatum* to prepare a beverage as a folk-treatment for cancer.[24] In Chinese folk-medicine the same *Ganoderma* has been applied in the treatment of cancer of the esophagus.

"Erroneously or not, it is believed that only specimens growing on the large-hooked honey-locust tree (*Gleditsia macrocantha* Desf.)," Ken paused to glance at his notes, "are efficacious in this application. Taken two to three times a day, a recipe calls for the stewing of 30 grams with the lungs and heart of a pig."[23]

"Not liable to be a popular dish over here," I interjected. "But what about research to back up the folklore?"

"Cancer research on the Ancient *Ling zhi* began in 1968. Researchers at the National Cancer Center Research Institute in Tokyo (Japan's equivalent of the National Cancer Institute of the U.S.) discovered that a water extract prepared from a specimen collected in the forests of Japan held antitumor activity comparable to the Shiitake mushroom (*Lentinus edodes*)."

> 50% of the cancerous tumors in mice completely regressed 10 days after injection of Reishi.

"Noting that in some parts of Japan the same fungus is a folk-treatment for cancer, one researcher reported that after daily injections in mice (200 mg/kg/day times ten days) tumors in 50% of the animals had completely regressed.[8]

"A later collaborative effort between the National Cancer Research Center and the Department of Agricultural Chemistry at Shizuoka University in Shizuoka, Japan in 1980 turned up one of the most potent polysaccharides of its kind. It was dubbed G-I-2a-*Beta*, the 'G-I' denoting Ganoderma Immunostimulant."[26]

> Even in small doses, a polysaccharide from Reishi inhibited 100% of tumors in mice.

"This polysaccharide is technically known as a *Beta*-D-Glucan. *Beta*-D-glucans are what hold together the cell walls of such cereal grains as barley, wheat and oats. The high potency of this polysaccharide was apparent in the rate at which it inhibited the formation of tumors - 100% from as little as 1 mg/kg in a single dose and in five out of five mice.[26]

"The scientists in this case found all the mice showed complete regressions of tumors (Sarcoma 180), even 20 days after the treatment period had ended. Curiously, 10 mg/kg was equally effective, but at 3 mg/kg just three out of five mice survived, which is, however, still a good rate, but at 0.3 mg/kg only two out of five survived. Further studies in Japan uncovered comparable and better results with a variety of polysaccharides from *Ganoderma*."[25,27]

"Dose-dependency again. Have the Japanese actively undertaken research on Reishi as well as more exotic extracts from it?" I asked.

"Right. By 1977, one team reported four polysaccharide preparations derived from Reishi (*G. lucidum*) had completely cured 50% of mice and without toxic effects.[10] Since then, a storm of research has issued from the Orient reporting antitumor results from more clearly defined isolates, either polysaccharides alone or protein-bound forms which are made up of amino acids and long-chain sugars.[1,10-68]

"For example, very significant results were reported in 1981 out of two Tokyo research labs who together had described a water-soluble polysaccharide they dubbed `GL-I.' From 20 mg/kg (for ten days), tumors in four out of five mice completely regressed."

"Once again," I said, "lots of mouse studies, lots of different extracts, but is there anything relating to humans apart from Morishige's work?"

"It's in the works I'd say," responded Ken. "Anticipating the potential utilization of Reishi polysaccharide preparations in human cancer, dramatic results against cancer in animal experiments led more than one Japanese corporation to patent the use."

> Confidence in Reishi has stimulated patent applications.

Referring to his notes, he read, "In 1982 a patent was granted to the Teikoko Chemical Industry Co., Ltd. for the application of *Ganoderma* glycoproteins as inhibitors in tumor formation.[20] As early as 1968 the Kureha Chemical Industry Co. Ltd. had applied for and later (1976) received patent approval for the application of a polysaccharide-containing powder derived from water extracts of *Ganoderma tsugae* Murril and *Ganoderma boninense* Pat. mycelia as an anticarcinogen.[21] A concentrated extract of *G. tsugae* (200 mg/kg) produced a tumor inhibition rate of 77.8% with 20% of mice completely cured."[22]

"Well, it's promising." I took a break to stand up and stretch, thinking about what Ken had said over the past hour or so. It was still a bit iffy though — research with mice and anecdotes with seriously ill people. It was a story I had heard so many times before. And yet the correspondence between the folk-literature and the scientific studies was undeniable.

The sun came flooding in from the windows overhead and reminded me of my conversation with Dr. Wu about vital energy — how Reishi seemed to revitalize the body in an almost mystical way. Yes, there were specific chemical reactions which could be traced. Yet the most striking evidence related to Reishi's ability to stimulate vital energy or *Wei Qi*. But how could I fit the biochemical information together with the anecdotes and experiences of Oriental healers?

We have seen that if injected, an extract of Reishi induces interferon production, thereby interfering with viral infection. It also inhibits bacteria. Long chain sugars called polysaccharides modulate the immune system while increasing bone marrow RNA and DNA. Reishi can also be shown to augment IgG and memory T-cells.

In the case of cancer, Reishi has shown long-term success. It has been shown to wake up the immune system to help fight cancer. In mice studies some of the chemicals have resulted in 50 - 100% regression rates on cancerous tumors. The Japanese Government lists Reishi as an official drug to use as a associated remedy for cancer. Research in this area has even stimulated patent applications.

I could see that there were direct indications for me to use it clinically. Time would tell how it worked in a clinical setting. I definitely decided to use it in wider clinical applications. Reishi certainly fit into the ancient concept of *Fu Zheng* therapy, adding it to the list of Echinacea, Siberian Ginseng, *Astragalus* and *Ligustrum*. That part of Dr. Wu's conversation was easy to confirm.

Chapter 4

Reishi and the Heart

It does seem that we can be quite confident that Reishi is a *Fu Zheng* herb that has specific as well as wide-spectrum immune modulating features. It is easy to say that in its process of enhancing the immune system, it also builds *qi* (from the perspective of Oriental medical theory)," I said.

"We can go further to say that it builds a specific type of *qi* called *wei qi* (protection *qi*). This *wei qi* is also known from an Oriental point of view to both protect the body from attacks of organisms and from the occurrence of cancer. It can also actively destroy cancer cells. Reishi has demonstrated a link to all of these factors in laboratory animals, test tubes and human anecdotal case histories.

"I think we are getting somewhere, Ken. The idea that Reishi will influence *wei qi* is quite exciting. The scientific evidence certainly does give credence to the myths about Reishi and *qi*.

"In Oriental philosophy there are many kinds of *qi*. The basic type of *qi*, the one related to vitality, `spiritual essence,' flows through the bloodstream. It is the essence of life. *Wei Qi* is considered to be on the outside of the blood vessels, surrounding them, kind of like a military protection.

"Let's look at Reishi's influence on the other type of *qi*, Ken, the one that flows through the body. Reishi is reported to work on the blood system in some of the papers I received from Jeff Chilton. Let's look at that area next."

As Ken went off with a new list of research items in hand, I started to think about the possible clinical application of the information that we had already assembled. I had several patients that could benefit from this herb immediately.

We hadn't yet shown Reishi to be the herb of *spiritual* potency, immortality or longevity, but we could certainly see its potential as a practical help for some people.

In response to my trips to the Orient and my reading and meetings with Ken and Jeff, I had already begun to integrate Reishi to a limited degree in my two clinics. Based on this meeting with Ken, I began to take the herb myself and to use it professionally in earnest.

A few weeks later I was back in British Columbia and arranged for another session with Ken. This time we focused on what he had found regarding Reishi's influence on the circulatory system. Was there evidence that it functioned significantly at this level?

The results were astonishing.

"I'd have to say that Reishi's effects on heart or blood-related conditions is as extensive as any of the other categories I've seen," Ken began. "Reishi remains true to its indications in the medical works of the Ming Dynasty, where the fungus called *chi zhi* or red fungus was prescribed to patients with tight or "knotted" chest and was said to positively affect the heart ch'i."[Chp.1 Notes, Ben Cao]

Reishi reduces blood fat levels, including "bad" cholesterol.

"Take this study as an example. Seventy patients suffering from hyperlipidemia — an elevated concentration of fats (lipids) and cholesterol in the blood plasma — were carefully screened from a larger patient population for a series of clinical trials at the Third Hospital of Hong Qiao District in Tianjin, China. An extract of wild *Ganoderma* (equivalent to one gram of the fungus), combined with the bioflavonoid hesperidin (extracted from mandarin orange peel), was formulated into a convenient tablet taken two to three at a time, three times a day for one to three months.[1]

"Although no explanation was given in the report for the inclusion of hesperidin, it was most probably added to reduce the aggregation or clumping together of blood cells — a condition reportedly common in cases of hypertension[2,3] and an especially dangerous one if it accompanies coronary atherosclerosis.[4] It could also have been combined with Reishi to lower cholesterol and reduce atherosclerosis.[5]

"All the patients were over 30 years of age. Diets remained unchanged except for those judged to be overweight or eating a high calorie diet. These patients continued with their normal daily work, whereas those presenting complications were instructed to rest. The normal cholesterol level was determined as 140 to 250 mg/dl.[1]

"There is no doubt that LDL (Low Density Lipoprotein or 'bad' cholesterol) levels dropped, but unfortunately the report does not specify by how much. Nonetheless, in no group of patients was the cure rate below 69.2%. On average, 74.2% of the total patient population found their cholesterol levels restored to the normal range. In conclusion, the study found best results achieved in those patients who limited animal fats in their diet and exercised. However, even in some of those who didn't, definite improvements were seen in cholesterol levels."[1]

"So the research has led us back to China," I said, "only this time we're dealing with heart-related problems and the use of the raw herb."

"Here's another one," said Ken.

"In patients on the same dosage of Reishi tablets, LDL levels fell in 68% of patients after one to four months treatment. The report states that the higher the serum cholesterol before treatment, the greater the drop after. In other words, Reishi helped those most who needed it most."[6]

"Looks like a dependable pattern," I agreed.

"The study was specifically conducted to test the *Ganoderma* tablets in coronary heart disease," continued Ken. "*Ganoderma Shu Xin* tablets were administered to 103 patients in seven different hospitals in the Nanjing area. All Western medications were removed except for nitroglycerin, if and when needed. The majority of patients ranged from age 40 to 60 years with a history of coronary heart disease of over one year. To be `effective,' the treatment had to either completely resolve or `markedly' alleviate the symptoms and at the same time improve the ECG reading."[6]

Reishi improves 81.77% of heart disease patients in 9 Chinese hospitals.

"A tall order for success, yet except for the most serious cases, in which the fungus proved ineffective, Reishi came through with flying colors. Out of a final total of 90 cases from seven different hospitals, the *Ganoderma* treatment was effective on average in 81.77% of patients. The lowest level of treatment effectiveness was 66.7% of cases! Best results were found at the Nanjing Gulou Hospital where 93.3% of coronary patients markedly improved after one to four months on the tablets. In addition, some patients experienced improved appetites, better spirits and weight gain.[6]

"As for side-effects, only one patient had an upset stomach. Regular checkups monitoring side-effects found no other instances.[6]

"I've put together a table adapted from a report on the trial in China in 1977. It offers a less generalized view of *Ganoderma*'s action in coronary heart disease as a symptom-by-symptom account of the outcome."

Table One[6]:

Patients with Coronary Heart Disease presenting:	Percentage of patients *Ganoderma* effective in:
Arrhythmia	60.0%
Sensation of fullness in chest	90.4%
Headache and dizziness	86.7%
Weariness	77.8%
Cold extremities	73.9%
Breathing difficulty (short breath)	72.5%
Insomnia	77.8%
Angina pectoris	84.4%

"Similar studies in China during the 1970's found a *Ganoderma* syrup effective in coronary heart disease and hyperlipidemia. In one study, 14 cases out of 15 had LDL levels substantially decreased. In another, 72% of 92 patients found relief from chest-pain and 65% had fewer problems breathing and reduced tachycardia. Irregular heart rhythm was restored to normal in 20 out of 52 patients after injections of *Ganoderma* extract and another 13 showed improvement.

"Remarkably, benefits were obtained in coronary heart disease patients after less than a week's treatment. Moreover, in three patients with digitalis-induced heart irregularity, the extract provided a quick recovery."[7]

"Were all of these studies done on the fruiting body?" I asked.

> ## Mycelium of Reishi also found to be very effective.

"No," replied Ken, "other studies show significant action from the mycelium — the fine thread-like vegetative body.

"*Mycelial* or *culture* products of Reishi have shown promising results in tests by various clinics and hospitals in China[8] and more recently in Japan.

"Let's see here." Ken shuffled through his notes. "A freeze-dried powder made from Reishi mycelium cultured with soybeans was administered to patients with hyperlipidemia. After four months of twice daily drinking 30 grams dissolved in a cup of water (200 ml), serum cholesterol levels significantly decreased. In one example, a patient showed a drop of 60 mg/dl, at which point the blood cholesterol fell to normal (250 mg/dl).[9]

"A traditional soy-based recipe for the treatment of heart disease calls for drying the sliced mushroom and then grinding it to a powder. The soybeans are baked and ground. The two powders are mixed, three parts soy to one part Reishi and taken three times a day with hot (boiled) water, 9 to 15 grams each time.[10]

"I've also spotted some commercial activity in mainland China. Reishi's cardiotonic effects are widely recognized in products such as the *Heart Relaxant Tablet* or *Ling zhi Shuxin Pian*.

"Reishi heart tablets are available in many countries outside of China. One such product, sold in North American herb stores, carries an insert stating that the tablets are indicated in hyperlipidemia, hypertension, coronary heart diseases and `general weakness after long suffering.' The insert also states that the product complies with pharmaceutical requirements laid out in the Chinese Pharmacopoeia, 1977 edition.[10]

"Studies in China have also focused on refining their understanding about the action of Reishi on the heart. They've tried various products, and found that whether tinctures or extracts of the fruit body or mycelium, Reishi improves the circulation of the myocardium (the innermost muscle of the heart), increases blood flow and lowers oxygen consumption. Early efforts to determine the components involved in these cardiotonic activities pointed to alkaloids and polysaccharides.[8]

"Water solutions of Reishi fruit body and mycelium yielded a polysaccharide fraction with significant cardiotonic effects. In cats and dogs, injection (i.v.) of the alkaloid fraction of the mycelium produced a 62% increase in coronary flow. Oxygen consumption and coronary resistance were `markedly lowered.' In guinea pigs, experimentally-induced obstructed circulation in the heart (myocardial infarction) was improved after injections of the crude mushroom extract."[8]

"More animal studies?" I said.

In up to 48% of heart disease patients, Reishi caused a marked improvement and in up to 86% a general improvement. This included patients with elevated blood lipids.

"Yes," said Ken, "many more, but I'll limit them to highlights of research with Reishi.

"Following numerous experiments with animals (rats, cats, dogs, guinea pigs and rabbits), and over seven years of clinical studies in patients with hyperlipidemia and coronary heart disease, Chinese authorities were able to calculate some figures for Reishi's general efficacy in these conditions. Significant improvement was reported in 20 to 48% of patients with the treatment effectively improving 56 to 86% of the total patient population.[8]

"Reishi was notably effective in improving the flow of blood to the heart in 7.6% of patients and was somewhat effective in 42 to 94% of the total number of patients studied. Symptomatically, improvements varied. Examples were reduced pain above the heart, difficult breathing, edema, and the sensation of irregular or rapid heart beat (palpitation)."[8]

"So if it has that much effect on cholesterol, blood lipids and as a cardiotonic, it must also have quite an effect on blood pressure," I said.

"The story gets even better when you look at that side of it," he replied.

Reishi's Effect on Hypertension

Hypertension or high blood pressure is one of North America's biggest health problems. More than 15% of the population suffer from it. Untreated, a hypertensive patient is at great risk of developing disabling or fatal heart failure, or kidney failure at an early age. Hypertension is the most important risk factor predisposing a person to coronary and cerebral atherosclerosis.

> Reishi lowers high blood pressure.

"Animal studies going back to 1972 in China, using various *Ling zhi* preparations in different kinds of animals, demonstrated that intravenous injections produce a significant blood pressure lowering (hypotensive) action. A somewhat different effect in dogs may be due to dosage and route of administration. A percolated extract preparation injected (i.v.) into anesthetized dogs at relatively high doses (1 to 1.7 g/kg) at first reduced and then later increased blood pressure.[8] Rest assured, however, no such action is reported from oral use of the mushroom in normal doses in hypertensive people,[11] nor in hypertensive animals fed the fungus.[12]

"In Japan in 1988, a scientific team compared the blood pressure and cholesterol levels of two groups of spontaneously hypertensive rats. One group was fed an ordinary diet supplemented with egg protein (10%). The other group received the same diet with the egg protein plus 5% of their total feed consisting of powdered Reishi mycelium which was grown in a medium consisting partly (2%) of soybean powder.[12]

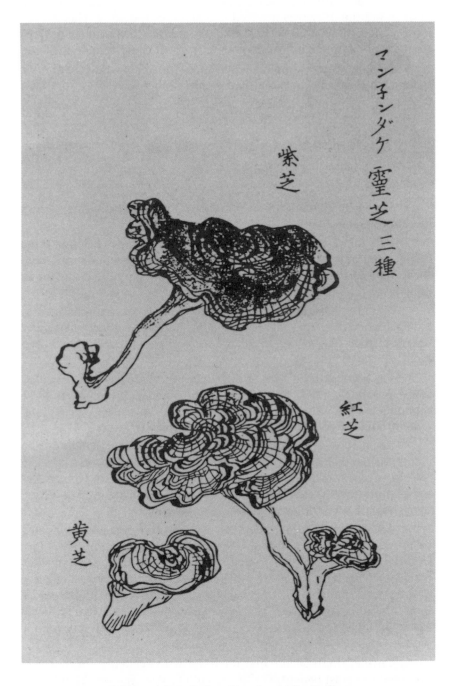

マンネンダケ 靈芝 三種

紫芝

紅芝

黄芝

Reishi mushrooms by Song Dynasty artist Zen-Yu Chen
from his book on mushrooms "Jun Pu". (repro: Hadeler)

"After four weeks the results showed that compared to the hypertensive rats without Reishi in their diet, total cholesterol in the blood plasma and the liver was lowered to a significant degree. This is even more significant when we consider that compared to normotensive rats, this type of rat has significantly greater levels of cholesterol in the liver.

"Finally, whereas heart rate was about the same in the two groups, those with Reishi in their diet had significantly lower blood pressure (systolic)."[12]

> ## You don't have to gorge yourself on Reishi to lower blood pressure.

"Similar results are found in humans and thankfully they didn't have to consume so much Reishi!

"Two things jump out right away about this study. The first is the phenomenal amount of Reishi powder the animals consumed relative to their body weight per day — equivalent to about a pound a day for an adult human.

"Usually, large amounts of plant materials are administered to animals when the experimenters are after noticeable effects. That way they don't have to wait long to go probing for the compounds that caused them.

"The second thing here is the soybean powder, which provided soybean saponins (530 mg/100 g Reishi powder).[12] In Japan these saponins are known to be clinically effective' in treating obesity and hyperlipidemia, both contributors to hypertension.[13]

"In animals, soybean saponins prevented blood platelets from clumping together in clots or forming `thrombi,'[13] which as we know can lead to stroke. However, according to my calculations, the amount of soyasaponin the rats consumed was sufficiently small (0.5 mg/kg/day)[12] to have made no significant difference to the results.

"A six month clinical trial of Reishi with 53 patients was conducted in Japan in 1984 in collaboration with the Asahi Chemical Industry Ltd. In order to establish some comparative results in hypertension, they placed patients with genetically inherited or `essential' hypertension in group one and patients with normal blood pressure or mild hypertension in group two. Patients were each given a supply of freeze-dried Reishi extract in tablet form, six 240 mg tablets to be taken each day for 180 days.[11]

"Once again, it seems that for those who needed it most, Reishi provided the most benefit. For the essential hypertensives, blood pressure was found to have `significantly decreased,' but not so for group

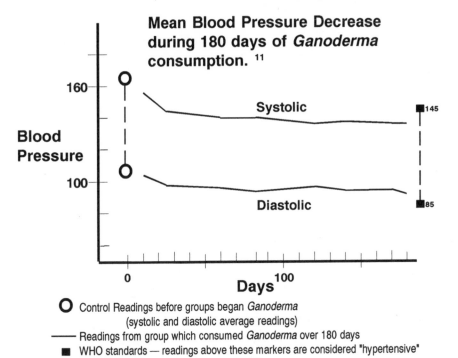

Mean Blood Pressure Decrease during 180 days of *Ganoderma* consumption. [11]

O Control Readings before groups began *Ganoderma*
(systolic and diastolic average readings)
—— Readings from group which consumed *Ganoderma* over 180 days
■ WHO standards — readings above these markers are considered "hypertensive"
(Adapted from Katsuo Kanmatsuse et al.[11])

two. Compared to the control blood pressure (BP) reading of 135.6 (systolic) over 92.5 (diastolic), only the systolic readings showed any significant change and then only occasionally. Changes were most noticeable at intervals of 25 days, again at 120 days and finally at the end of the treatment period (180 days) when the mean BP was 126.4/91."[11]*

> Significant reduction in blood pressure was noted in humans after taking Reishi tablets for 10 days.

"As for the essential hypertensives, 10% had systolic blood pressure decreases from 20 to 29 mm Hg. (= millimeters of mercury) and 47.5% had decreases of from 10 to 19 mmHg. Diastolic BP decreased by 10 to 14

---

* Systolic pressure is the blood pressure exertion gauged from the brachial artery which is located in the upper arm. This represents a reading of the blood pressure during the contraction or pumping phase of the heart. When the heart expands or relaxes before the next pump, the pressure being exerted in the brachial artery is called the diastolic pressure.

61

mmHg in 17.5% and by 5 to 9 mmHg in 42.5%. The mean drop in BP for the essential hypertensives was significantly different from the control at every point tested after the first ten days on Reishi, and this appeared in both systolic and diastolic pressures.[11]

"Compared to the mean BP of the control (156.6/103.5), which represented the BP of the patients in group one before treatment and which is well within World Health Organization standards for 'essential' hypertension — 165.5 (plus or minus 18.9) over 106.4 (plus or minus 11 mmHg). The mean BP score for group one (genetically inherited hypertension) 10 days before the end of the six month trial—136.6/92.8—came closer to the WHO standard for normal blood pressure.[11]

"One other benefit, though slight, is worth mentioning. In both groups of patients at the end of the trial there was in addition a decrease in 'total' cholesterol — from a mean total of 216.2 (plus or minus 48 mg/dl) at the start of the trial to 201 (plus or minus 32 mg/dl) at the end. It is significant that their HDL (High Density Lipoproteins or 'good' cholesterol) didn't change, which means the good cholesterol remained while the unwanted LDLs decreased. This is the ideal way to lose cholesterol. It is also the reason why the now popular rice and oat bran work."

"Do we know what the mechanism is, Ken?" I asked.

"It looks like the major mechanism lies in the Reishi's triterpenes," Ken said.

Triterpenes and Sterols

"Components of the mushroom known as 'triterpenes' are responsible for Reishi's bitter taste and several of its medicinal properties.[14,15] (See Appendix on Triterpenes and Sterols.)

"Investigators in China noted in 1986 that the mycelium of Reishi is rich in triterpenes and in sterols, both quantitatively and in terms of variety.[31] Naturally, *G. applanatum* (the Ancient *Ling zhi*) contains sterols too.[29,30,32,33]

> Triterpenes seem to be the component responsible for blood pressure and blood lipid improvements.

"One American authority on Chinese herbology, Subhuti Dharmananda, Ph.D., has noted that plants containing appreciable amounts of sterols, closely related steroids and steroid-like triterpenes, such as Reishi and *Panax ginseng*, are typically used as longevity herbs. They are applied in much the same conditions that steroidal hormones would be in Western medicine, including impotence and inflammation."[34]

> Triterpenes give Reishi an adaptogenic quality, providing the person with protection from a wide range of biological, environmental and social stresses.

"In short, these triterpenes seem to have an adaptogenic effect, helping the body to adapt to a large range of environmental, biological, and sociological stress. They have a kind of a harmonizing effect on the body. These harmonizing effects are on the immune system as well as the circulatory system.

"The vast majority of triterpenoids in Reishi occur as fatty acids called `lucidenic" and `ganoderic' acids.[41] The occurrence of each of the many types identified varies from strain to strain and from one growth stage of the fungus to the next in both the fruit body and the mycelium. It looks as though the major triterpenoids of *G. lucidum* mycelium (cultured) are the ganoderic acids R, S, and T.[42]

"The sterols in *Ganoderma* are of the `lanosterol' and `ergosterol' types, the latter becoming vitamin D_2 when exposed to ultraviolet irradiation. Sterols are components of membranes and also act as hormone precursors.[43] They are widely distributed in nature as alcohols occurring in both the animal and plant kingdoms.

"Sterols are structurally related to some of the sex hormones in animals and to bile acids. For example, cholesterol is an animal sterol that through a natural process of conversion in the body becomes bile acids and steroidal hormones. At an earlier stage in the process, cholesterol forms through the conversion of lanosterol.[44]

"However, although containing lanosterols, Reishi does not increase bile acids,[45] and as previously discussed, lowers cholesterol.

" As you can see, sterols are the `parents' of steroids. Pharmaceutical companies take advantage of this fact. For example, sitosterol, a major plant sterol we've all consumed, has been extracted to manufacture adrenal and steroidal hormones and hydrocortisone.[44]

" `Beta-sitosterol', another of the major plant sterols, inhibits tumor growth[46] and formation. This sterol, among the myriad other tumor-inhibitors found in plants, may be the key to why vegetarians have lower incidences of cancer affecting the colon."[47]

Anti-Hypertensive Triterpenes

"In China, cardiotonic activity[8] from Reishi was ascribed to undefined polysaccharides and alkaloids. Similarly, undefined high molecular weight substances showed anti-hypertensive activities in Japanese studies.[48]

"These early findings may yet hold true, but a number of scientists had mentioned that among the triterpenes isolated from Reishi were several having structures akin to sterols known for their ability to lower cholesterol.[31,49]

"In 1988, it was announced that potent inhibitors of cholesterol biosynthesis had been successfully isolated in Japan. Only a weak action was observed with the natural derivative triterpene, ganoderic acid B. Several further derivatives were chemically converted from the original, and as well, from ganoderic acid C. They proved very active inhibitors of cholesterol biosynthesis.[50]

"Nonetheless, many other triterpenes in the mushroom have similar structures with key placements of oxygen common to the cholesterol biosynthesis-inhibiting derivatives.[50] In fact, in the same year investigators in China found two more cholesterol-biosynthesis inhibitors in the mycelium of Reishi called ganoderic acid Mf and ganodermic acid T-O."[70]

Reishi contains over 100 triterpenes.

"Because certain triterpenes may account for multiple activities of Reishi, considerable time and effort has gone into their isolation and chemical elucidation. Currently, about 100 different triterpenoids are known to occur in either the fruit body or the mycelium of *G. lucidum*, or both. Only a handful have undergone bio-activity studies, but it is known that at least eight have a distinct anti-hypertensive action.

"In 1985, researchers at the Asahi Brewery Co., Ltd. in Tokyo, in collaboration with the Tokyo Institute of Technology, isolated eight active triterpenes from a methanol extract of the fruit body.[48] They also demonstrated anti-hypertensive activity with triterpenes from Reishi in spontaneously hypertensive rats."[51]

Some of Reishi's influence on blood pressure is attributable to ACE inhibition, an activity common to some pharmaceutical drugs.

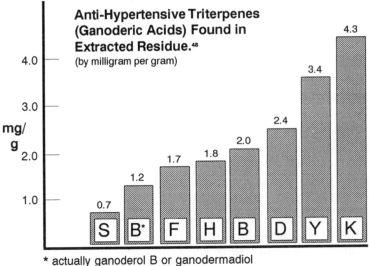

Anti-Hypertensive Triterpenes
(Ganoderic Acids) Found in
Extracted Residue.[48]
(by milligram per gram)

* actually ganoderol B or ganodermadiol

The relative proportion of Ganoderic Acids in Reishi

"The anti-hypertensive action of these triterpenes is mediated through the inhibition of an enzyme known as the `angiotensin converting enzyme' or ACE.[48] ACE inhibitors, though a relatively new type of drug treatment for high blood pressure, have gained wide acceptance in Western medicine for the simple reason that they work when all others have failed. And they work most expediently."[52,53]

"So there are some immediate practical benefits from these plant derivatives for modern medicine?" I asked.

"Because ACE-inhibitors are so effective," Ken replied, "pharmacologists are hard at work developing safer ones.[55] Although it's too soon to tell, the possibility of a triterpenoid ACE-inhibitor, perhaps from Reishi, does exist. As for the mushroom, while not presenting side-effects, it is slower-acting against hypertension[11] and apparently not effective in advanced cases of coronary heart disease.[6]

"Whether Reishi alone can reverse, reduce or prevent left ventricular hypertrophy, who knows? I haven't spotted it in the literature yet."

"Sounds good, Ken, but all of this is from a Western scientific point of view. Do we have any research that can show us a little more about the *qi* aspect of this herb?" I asked.

Reishi alleviates "bad blood" or *qi* deficient blood (*Oketsu*)

"The Japanese have been studying an ancient concept called *Oketsu* (bad blood), or *qi*-deficient blood. This concept is hard to tie down in Western terms, but after much investigation the Japanese government now covers it under the Japanese National Health care.

"Reishi is a herb that can deal with bad or *qi*-deficient blood. Since it is able to dislodge `blockages' in the body it is particularly appropriate for *Oketsu* therapy and is used extensively in Japan for this purpose."

"It seems the Japanese are somewhat more open-minded on this subject than North Americans," I said.

"Yes," he replied. "The Japanese have been really active in the study of herbal materials from a traditional perspective. It's interesting to note that in traditional Chinese medicine, myocardial infarction is equivalent to `stagnated blood in the heart' while pain is interpreted as `stagnant *qi*.'

"In Osaka, pharmaceutical scientists investigated the effects of Reishi on blood coagulation and platelet aggregation in 1983. Coagulated blood was experimentally induced in the vascular system of rats by way of `endotoxin,' a toxic lipopolysaccharide from bacterial cell walls.[56]

"For the purpose of comparing strains, water extracts of Reishi were prepared from samples of Reishi collected in Odawara and in Kyoto, some 200 miles away.[56]

"For the sake of further comparison, other groups received various doses of aspirin[56] — a well-known inhibitor of platelet aggregation and one that's been tested for reducing heart attacks.[59]

"Large doses of Reishi and of aspirin were employed in order to quickly obtain readings significantly different from controls. At 500 mg/kg, the Kyoto strain was not only significantly active, it was impressively more effective than the 50 mg/kg dose of aspirin. This was measured in terms of restoring to normal the number of platelets circulating in the blood and in coagulation factors such as the amount of fibrinogen and fibrin degradation products. Additional measurements were taken of the amounts of time the blood clotting protein prothrombin acted in coagulating the blood. The latter two measurements were restored very close to normal by Reishi.[56]

"A tougher test for Reishi was devised with the endotoxin-induced coagulation in rats fed so much butter they developed elevated levels of cholesterol and fats called `triglycerides.' This time neither strain of Reishi produced any significant changes in the blood except for lowering cholesterol, at which task the Odawara strain was the more active Reishi in the same doses (500 and 1000 mg/kg)."[56]

Reishi inhibits platelet aggregation.

"Finally, it was demonstrated that Reishi has a direct action against platelet aggregation. In the `test tube,' 500 to 1000 micrograms of Reishi/ml of blood with either strain produced an inhibitory action on platelets induced to aggregate by the platelet aggregation inducers collagen and thrombin.[56]

"A few years later, scientists at the prestigious Tokyo Institute of Technology isolated the platelet aggregation inhibitor itself. A water-soluble extract of Reishi proved active in an `incubation time-dependent' fashion, which may be why no one had previously isolated the active constituent.[57]

"If Reishi was first left to incubate with blood at 37°C (98.6°F) for two minutes, when thrombin was added the degree of platelet aggregation inhibition was higher than when the incubation period was only one minute. Allowed to incubate for six minutes, the degree of inhibition was approximately seven times that of a one minute incubation.[57]

"Next, they tried to find the limits of the action. One hundred times they diluted extract, but still it showed significant inhibitory action. Since they had apparently observed activity from as little as a single microliter of the active fraction of the Reishi extract, the researchers recognized that whatever this substance might be it was obviously potent."

One of the physical reservoirs for *qi* might be adenosine.

"In the end they would determine beyond any doubt that the inhibitor was a nucleotide, a derivative of RNA known as adenosine. Furthermore, they established that at the very least, adenosine occurs in the dried fungus on the order of 400 micrograms/gram.[57]

"Adenosine has been connected with the inhibition of platelet aggregation. It's the core of cyclic AMP and ATP, the basic communication and energy systems of our body." (See Appendix for a discussion of adenosine.)

"Ken, could the chemical adenosine, in its cAMP and ATP form, be a chemical component for the Chinese concept of *qi*?"

"Perhaps so. Adenosine is released in all kinds of psychological stress and is produced by the heart when the blood supply is down. It also seems to have an analgesic effect.

"I can't help but wonder how the old Taoists seemed to know this all along. Remember what it said in that medical text from the 16th century?"

"Here it is," Ken said. "The document says that the Red or Chi-fungus (*chi zhi*) was prescribed to patients who had tight or `knotted' chest and that it would positively affect the `heart ch'i' or its `energy' and that it would `mend the chest.' If that doesn't describe heart disease or angina, I don't know what does, Terry."

"Ken, the pieces are starting to come together. This is some herb here!"

"Indeed. We have matching evidence from mainland China."

Reishi contributes to pain relief.

"In the 1970s, for example, a concentrated extract of *Ling zhi* showed analgesic activity in mice regardless of oral intake or injected administration (i.p.). In rats, a non-concentrated extract demonstrated significant pain-relieving action. In addition, for 90% of chronic bronchitis patients treated with various preparations of the mushroom for a period of four months, blood analysis indicated that parasympathetic nervous system excitability was reduced. A `knotted chest' may pertain here, too.[8]

Reishi has a calming effect.

"Even in the absence of records specifying the use, I suspect this famous mushroom of longevity may have served some function as an aid to meditation. Perhaps it was even used to promote mind over body transmutations, either real or imagined. The instructions for such a use are probably lost in antiquity or remain in some dusty document no one has ever bothered to decipher.

"Then again, the calming effect of the mushroom may have simply been a fortuitous part of monastic life in the pursuit of harmony with nature. What is certain though is that the attainment of tranquility remains as inseparable from the purpose of the alchemists who held Reishi in such high regard in the past as it is from the subject of longevity and heart disease today."

I sat back in my chair and thought about the remarkable thing we had been discussing. Problems in the cardiovascular area represent four of the top five killing ailments in North America. Reishi certainly has shown some very significant therapeutic value in this area.

The mass media are constantly telling us about how we need to reduce our cholesterol and blood-fat levels. Not only has Reishi been shown to do this, it also balances the ratio of good cholesterol to bad cholesterol. In fairly exhaustive studies Reishi has been shown to help over 80% of people with, heart problems. This research confirmed the classical statement of Reishi's use for "knotted chest."

Blood pressure, a big problem with patients I see, is dramatically lowered in as little as 10 days. It appears that the triterpenes are as significant here as the polysaccharides. Reishi's effect on blood pressure may work through the same mechanism used by some pharmaceuticals, that of ACE-inhibition.

The Oriental concept of 'bad blood' or *Oketsu*, is not completely foreign to Western herbology. It was heavily used in the last century, as much by medical doctors as by herbalists. This idea fits in very well with some of my own concepts of aging. Reishi's effect in this area really added support in my mind to its reputed ability to slow down the aging process.

Platelet aggregation has been a big topic in the 80s. Here too, Reishi has shown inhibiting effects. By inhibiting platelet aggregation, the incidence of problems such blood clots, stroke and migraine can be lowered.

The idea of adenosine functioning on *qi* is something that certainly deserves more attention. Reishi's ability to calm the body and regulate its energy seems to be the key to its effect on blood pressure, the immune system, and ultimately how long that system will last.

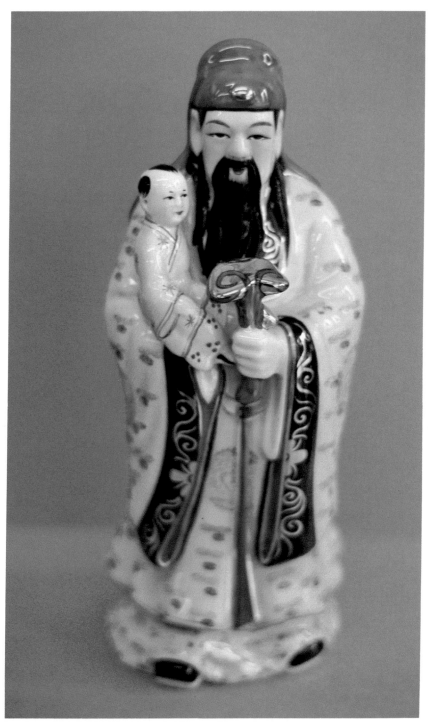

1. Chinese sage holding the Ling zhi. (Photo: Chilton)

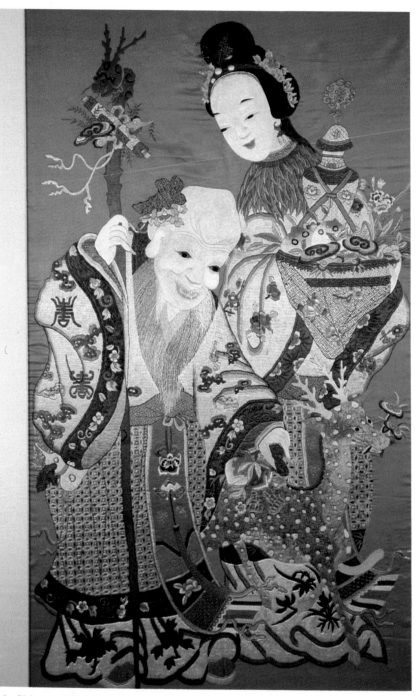

2. Chinese silk tapestry, pre-1940. Immortal of Longevity and Princess. Reishi mushrooms depicted in deer's mouth, basket, and on the staff. (courtesy of Coleman Luthie. Photo: Francine Katz)

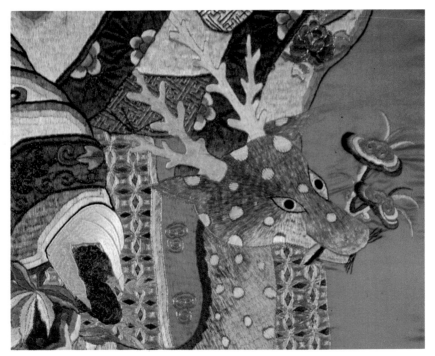

3. Association of antlered deer and Reishi. (Photo: Francine Katz)

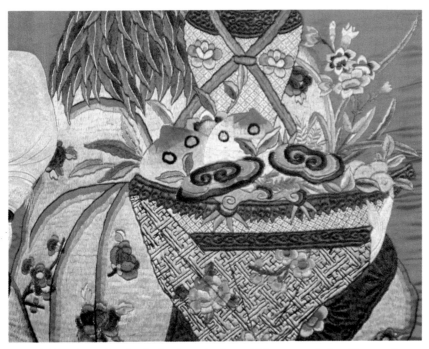

4. Reishi and peaches in the basket-- both are Chinese symbols of longevity.
   (Photo: Francine Katz)

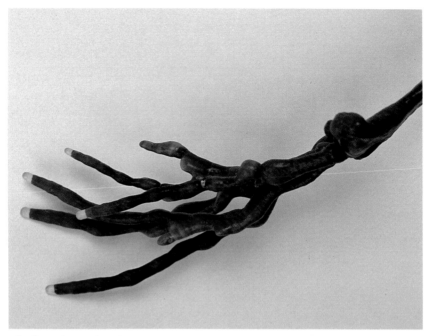

5. *Ganoderma lucidum*, antler form. Yellow tips are the newest growth.
(Photo: Hadeler)

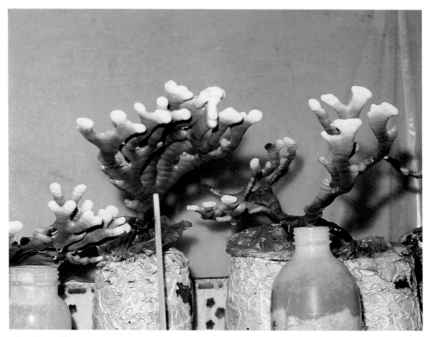

6. *Ganoderma tsugae*, antler form, growing in sterilized sawdust media.
(Photo: Hseu)

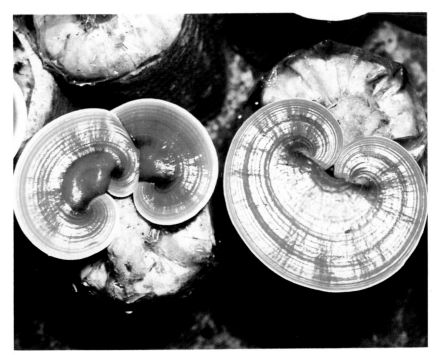

7. *Ganoderma lucidum* growing on sterilized sawdust media. (Photo: Hseu)

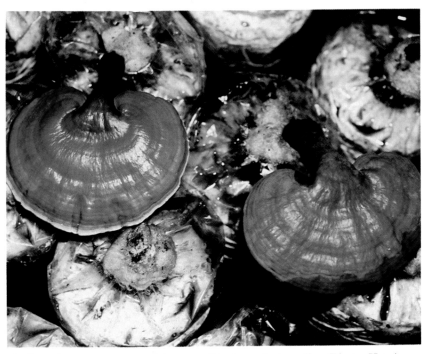

8. *Ganoderma tsugae* growing on sterilized sawdust media. (Photo: Hseu)

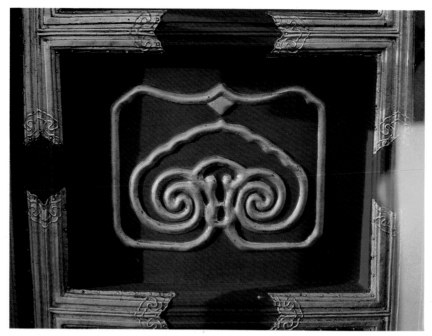

9. Reishi motif on a pavillion door in the Forbidden City, Beijing.
   (Photo: Chilton)

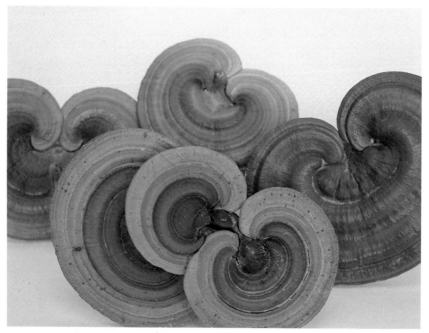

10. Red Reishi mushrooms. *Ganoderma lucidum.* Classic ram's horn
    shape. (Photo: Hadeler)

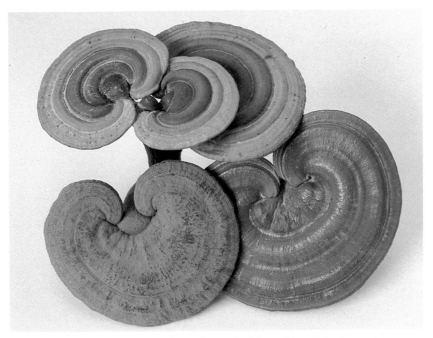

11. Red Reishi mushrooms -- *Ganoderma lucidum*. Unpolished cap at bottom left shows a coating of brown spores. (Photo: Hadeler)

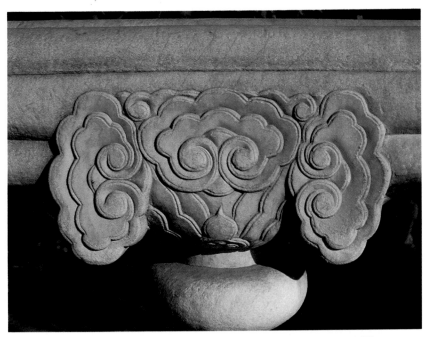

12. Ram's horn or cloud form Reishi motif -- ubiquitous on stone railing supports in the Forbidden City, Beijing. (Photo: Chilton)

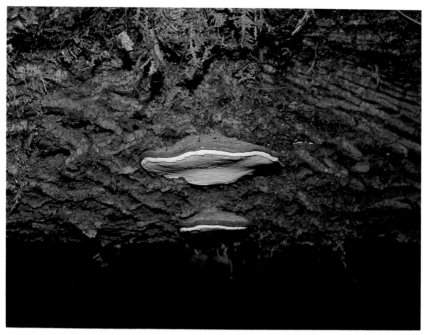

13. The Ancient Ling zhi, *Ganoderma applanatum*, growing wild in British
    Columbia. (Photo: Hadeler)

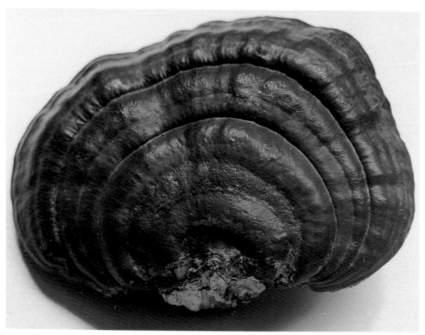

14. *Ganoderma oregonense*, one North American Reishi species.
    (Photo: Hadeler)

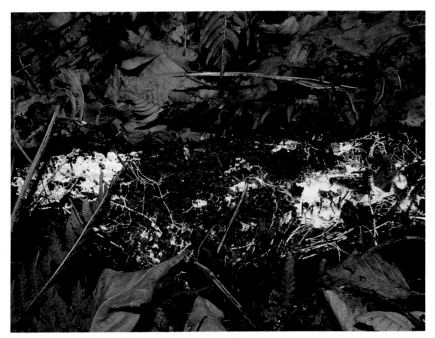

15. Reishi mushroom mycelium growing on wood in nature. (Photo: Hadeler)

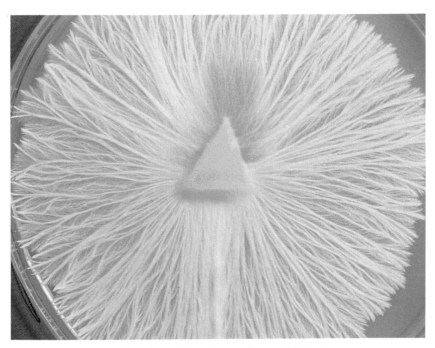

16. Mushroom mycelium in sterile culture. (Photo: Chilton)

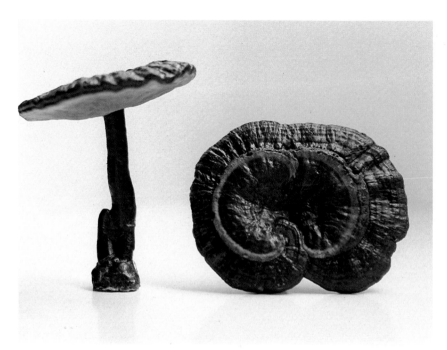

17. *Ganoderma sinense*. The Chinese black Reishi. (Photo: Hadeler)

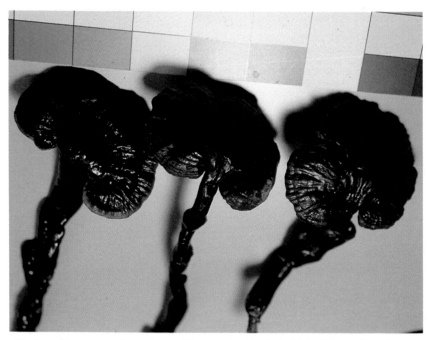

18. *Ganoderma neo-japonicum*. The purple-black Reishi. (Photo: Hseu)

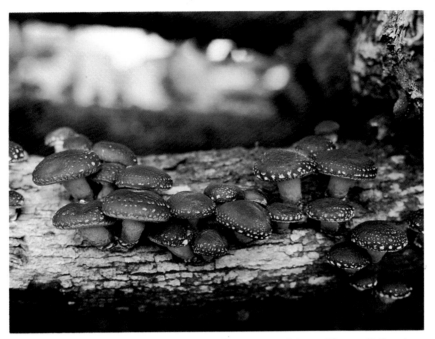

19. Cultivated shiitake mushrooms growing on an oak log. (Photo: Chilton)

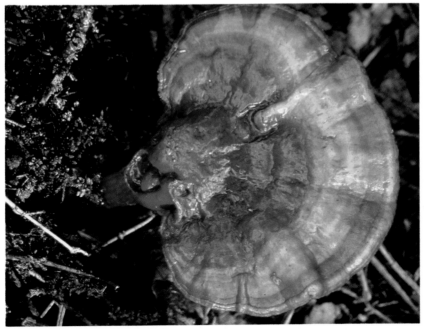

20. Wild European Reishi mushroom. *Ganoderma lucidum.*
    (Photo: J.H. Petersen)

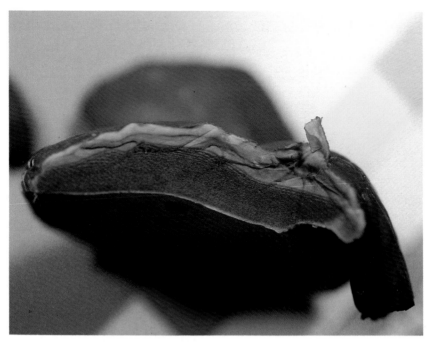

21. Cross section of a Reishi mushroom. Dark brown area is the pore layer. (Photo: Hseu)

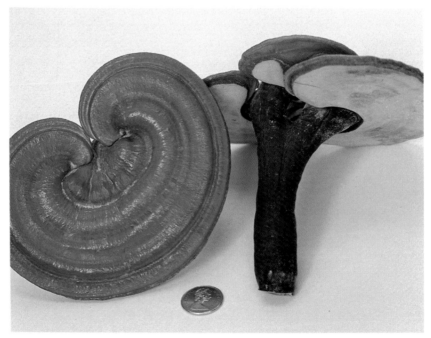

22. *Ganoderma lucidum*, cap surface and underside. Note light cream to yellow pore layer. (Photo: Hadeler)

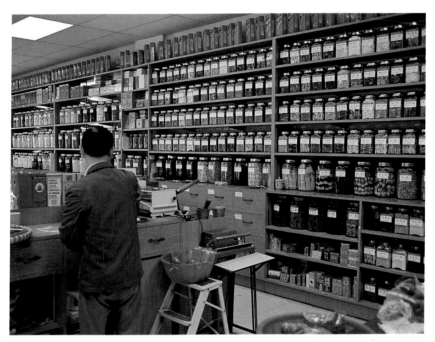

23. Contemporary Chinese herbal pharmacy, Vancouver, B.C.
    (Photo: Hadeler)

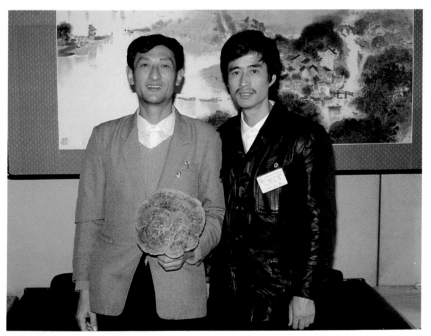

24. Chinese wild mushroom collectors showing off a giant Reishi.
    (Photo: Chilton)

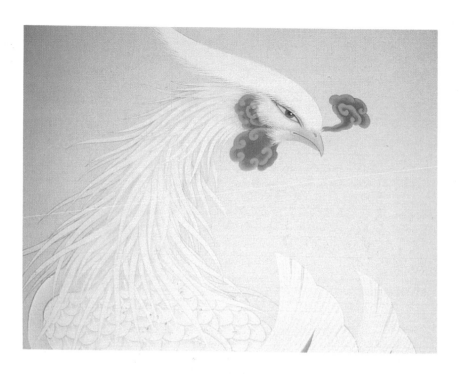

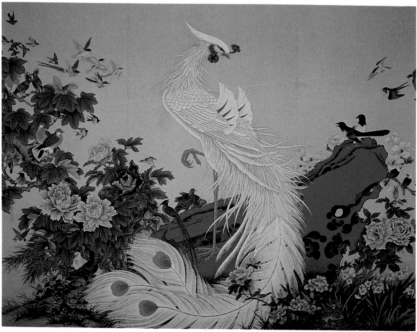

25,26. Contemporary Chinese painting depicting the Phoenix bird holding a Reishi mushroom in its beak. Both are ancient Chinese symbols of longevity. (Photos: Chilton)

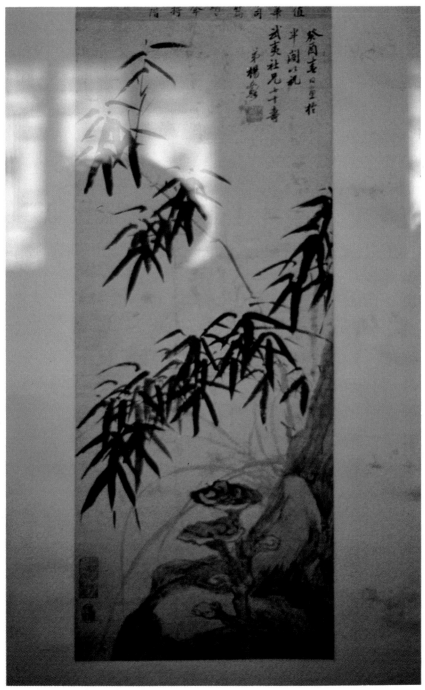

27. Bamboo, Stone, Ling zhi, and Green Grass, circa 1600. Given to the
   Emperor on his 70th birthday with wishes for good health and long life.
   In the art gallery of the Forbidden City, Beijing. (Photo: Chilton)

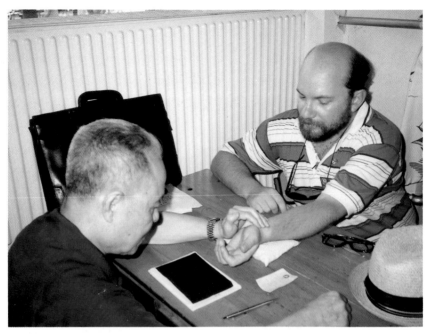

28. The author, Terry Willard, consulting with an herbalist to the Last Emperor of China.

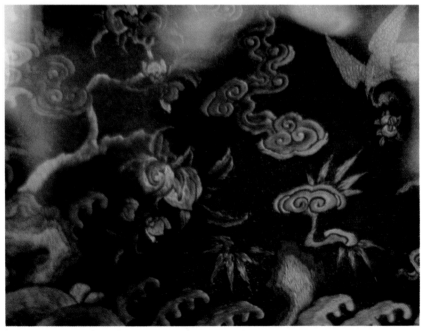

29. Peach tree, cloud forms, and Reishi, on the Chinese Emperor's finely embroidered silk robe. Forbidden City, Beijing. (Photo: Chilton)

Chapter 5

Reishi and The Issue of Allergies

When I've talked to some of my Oriental colleagues about Reishi over the past few months, one of the first things that comes up is its effect on allergic asthma. This should be our next area of investigation Ken," I said.

A few weeks later we were again back in a room reviewing stacks of photocopies. We took up our discussion in what was becoming the ritual of looking at the amazing powers of Reishi. Although I wasn't about to believe wholeheartedly in the ancient myths about Reishi, with the breadth and quality of the recent research material and the exciting results I had begun to see in my own practice, I was certainly developing a great respect for this herb.

It was easy to see why so much mysticism surrounded it. Without some of the scientific tools of the present day, the only explanation of how it worked so strongly on so many health problems was "magic." And I must admit, after taking this herb myself on a daily basis for several months, some of the magic was rubbing off on me.

The Anti-Allergic Aspect

"What do you have today Ken?" I asked.

> Reishi helps alleviate allergies.

"Another ailment — the application of Reishi in treating chronic bronchitis, a use believed centuries old. This knowledge recently led Japanese pharmacologists to inquire into the active constituents with the hope of finding a better means to combat the unprecedented incidence of allergies currently plaguing the industrialized world.[37,38]

"From clinical assessments in China during the 1970's, it was a fairly safe bet that an investigation of Reishi for anti-allergic substances would turn up something. In over 2,000 case studies of chronic bronchitis in various hospitals and clinics, individuals were treated with a tabletted form of Reishi syrup."[1]

Reishi provided relief to 60-90% of chronic bronchitis sufferers. Older patients experienced greater relief.

"In most cases, dramatic effects were seen within the first two weeks. Appetite and the overall condition of the patients noticeably improved. Historically and pharmacologically, it is interesting that the aged should show the most improvement. After all, Reishi has been regarded as a geriatric medicine since ancient times. Adding up the successes and failures, the overall rate of effectiveness has been calculated at 60 to 90% of the cases."[1]

Ken's comments would mean little unless you know a little about how allergies occur and the role of the chemical histamine. The release of histamine in allergic reactions, which causes the familiar redness and swelling responses of tissues, also causes smooth muscles to contract, particularly those in the bladder, gastrointestinal tract, uterus and bronchi — the big air ducts in our lungs which are interlaced with smooth muscles.[40]

Constriction of the bronchi results in the typical breathing difficulty or 'asthmatic attack' of the hay fever sufferer. In addition, the release of histamine in the gastrointestinal tract in allergic responses to foods can cause diarrhea. Histamine also stimulates the secretion of bronchial mucus, tears, saliva and gastric secretions,[40] so the more obvious action of a potential anti-allergic agent would be the inhibition of histamine release, which is exactly what pharmacologists in Japan hoped to find with Reishi.

Reishi inhibits histamine release.

Ken continued, "Important work preceded them in China, where it was already established that a Reishi extract caused a marked inhibition of histamine release in sensitized guinea pig lung tissue subjected to foreign substances that trigger immune responses called 'antigens.' The more Reishi administered, the more histamine release was inhibited. Other experiments in China found Reishi preparations relaxed smooth muscles induced to constrict by histamine.[1] Reishi also strongly inhibited chemically-induced uterine contractions in rat uteruses.[1]

"Without determining their precise nature, pharmacologists at Beijing Medical College had determined that the most obvious active constituents in Reishi were 'acid substances.'[1]

"In 1985, a Japanese university-industry consortium headed by Mori Nogami, using a particular strain of Reishi dubbed 'No. 9,' determined that in rodents given a large oral dose of the fruit body in the form of a water extract (500 mg/kg), the degree of various anti-allergic responses was significant, even remarkable.[41,42] Reishi showed a significant preventive activity in experimentally-induced asthma and contact dermatitis in guinea pigs, and notably inhibited the formation of kidney lesions from serum sickness nephritis. At the same time it decreased the excretion of protein into urine.[42]

"Reishi was put through more difficult tests. Nogami induced histamine release in the mast cells of rats using a chemical and in another experiment using antigen. Reishi came through again, significantly inhibiting the release of histamine by either inducing agent. The results of these and other tests indicated that Reishi has a definite effect on 'IgE-related' allergic reactions.[41]

"IgE antibodies mediate 'type I' hypersensitivities, the often dramatic severe inflammatory (anaphylactic) reactions to pollens, proteins and insect venoms, which require immediate application of anti-histamines. The allergic individual produces IgE in response to certain foreign proteins (antigens) or allergens but at an abnormally high rate. This is due to a lack of suppressor T-cells (which shut down the antibody response so it doesn't go on indefinitely and histamine release doesn't get out of hand).[40]

"With an abnormally high rate of IgE, an inordinate number of mast-cells are contacted with subsequent degranulation and histamine release. Coincidentally, cyclic nucleotides modulate mast-cell degranulation. If the level of cyclic AMP in mast-cells is raised, degranulation is inhibited.[40] What role Reishi plays at this level with its content of adenosine hasn't been worked out as far as I know. That applies as well to the anti-inflammatory role of Reishi as a potent scavenger of free radicals and modulator of T-cells. These actions may well contribute to its anti-allergic abilities in chronic bronchitis and perhaps in other similar kinds of applications.

"In 1984, Japanese researchers announced that they had managed to isolate ganoderic acids C_2 and D as two of the main histamine inhibitor/anti-inflammatory components of the Reishi mushroom. They added that ganoderic acid B[44] (also an anti-hypertensive)[42] and ganoderic acid A were active too, though not as potent as C_2 and D, with A being at least 50% less active.[44]

"Meanwhile, Mori Nogami's team was still at work at Kinki University with the No. 9 strain. In 1988, a member of the team travelled to the U.S. to present more recent results. At the International Congress on Natural Products Research, held in Park City, Utah, Masaaki Ito elaborated on their successful culture of a strongly anti-allergic strain of a mushroom known since ancient times as a life-elixir in the Orient, called Reishi."[38]

Reishi inhibits Type I, II, III, and IV allergic sensitivity reactions.

"Animal studies indicated the water extract of No. 9 strain not only inhibited allergic reactions in type I hypersensitivities, but also had shown strong anti-allergic effects against types II, III and IV hypersensitivity models. This proved Reishi has a wide range of anti-allergic activity. Dr. Ito added that with the increasing incidence of `intractable allergic diseases' fostered by a complexity of predisposing factors, a broad spectrum anti-allergic agent like Reishi had become something of a requirement. Speaking on behalf of his colleagues at home in Osaka, Dr. Ito conveyed their hope that in the very near future the mushroom would go beyond animal studies and be clinically applied in the treatment of patients with allergies.[38]

"The `Type II' hypersensitivity is seen in the inflammation resulting from `immune wars' when antibodies or cytotoxic immune cells (such as macrophages, NK cells and killer T-cells) seek out and attack viral, foreign and tumor cells. Type II is also called `cytotoxic hypersensitivity.'[47]

"Type III reactions are in response to an excess of antigens bound to antibodies. These antigens form `complexes' that macrophages have a difficult time removing. However, if antibodies are in excess in the complex, macrophages and other phagocytes process them efficiently. What happens is that these excess-antigen complexes deposit themselves inside of vessel walls. The result is acute inflammation, a type III reaction.[48]

"Extremely moldy hay contributes to a type III hypersensitivity reaction called `Farmer's lung.' An organism (actinomycete) grows in the hay leaving behind its tiny spores in massive quantities. If enough of these spores are inhaled, the onslaught of antibodies attacking them can lead to persistent `complexes.' Hoards of phagocytes come along to gobble up the mess, but they don't get it all the first time. The ones that get away, for the time being, can lodge themselves in the little air sacks of the lungs, predisposing the farmer to severe pneumonia.[49]

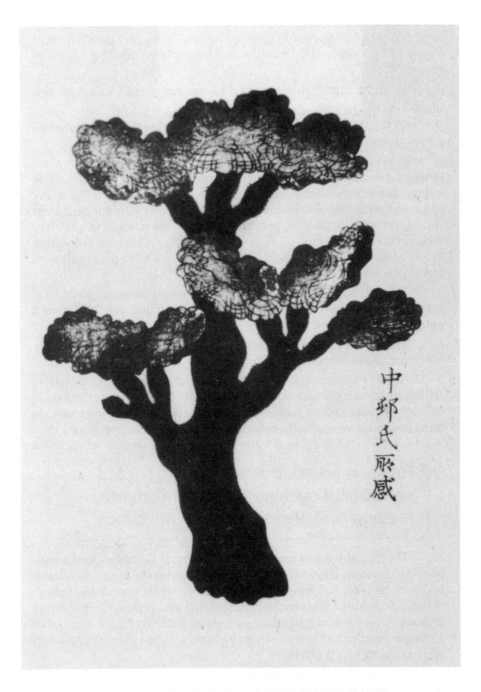

Reishi depiction from Sakikusa-ko, "An Inquiry into the Happy Herb"
by Suigetsu Kan-o, Japan, 1850. (repro: Hadeler)

"By the same process, people who write about medicinal fungi and often spend ridiculously long hours in libraries filled with old books, can develop `Librarian's lung,' a type III hypersensitivity reaction resulting from book-dust. `Mushroom growers disease' is another classic form of a type III hypersensitivity reaction and results from inhaling too many spores."[49]

"Is that a hint that you've picked up `Librarian's Lung' on this project, Ken?" I joked.

"You don't have to be worry about me," he laughed. "I take Reishi daily -- who wouldn't be by this stage of the research?

"Anyway, back to the material at hand. Reishi inhibits the lesions on kidneys caused by serum sickness nephritis. Not surprisingly, these lesions are immune-complex mediated. Again, the cause is too many antigens for the immune system to deal with at once. The antigens form complexes with antibodies and then deposit themselves in capillary walls, in the synovial fluid of joints and in arterial walls where, in addition to the attendant inflammation, they can stimulate the aggregation of blood platelets.[49]

"Type III reactions are common to autoimmune and chronic viral diseases,[49] lupus, and to rheumatoid arthritis, in which case IgM-bound antigens are deposited in joints.[50]

"I have some interesting material on these problems that I'll show you later," Ken interjected.

"Type IV hypersensitivity reactions are of the delayed kind characterized by contact dermatitis. These involve the activation of cytotoxic T-cells by antigens such as poison ivy.[51] Associated autoimmune reactions include ulcerative colitis, diabetes mellitus and myasthenia gravis."[50]

> ## Reishi is an aid in other immune-related sensitivities such as chronic pneumonia, rheumatism, hepatic disease and cancer.

"Dr. Morishige was among the first clinical witnesses to the antibody modulating effects of Reishi. He ran tests on the immunoglobulin levels of patients suffering from chronic bronchial pneumonia, rheumatic-autoimmune diseases, hepatic diseases and cancer. He found that in most of the immunoglobulin cases, those with too high a number of antibodies had reductions and those patients with too short a supply had their antibody levels increased.[52]

"Morishige noted that this included IgE antibodies,[52] the ones that mediate type I hypersensitivity reactions. Examples of Type I reactions are severe inflammatory responses to pollens and insect bites. This modulating effect acted also upon IgM, the major class of antibodies residing in the vascular system which mount the first line attack against cells infested with viruses and bacteria[53] and IgA, a deficiency of which is associated with the severest allergies.[54] This immunoglobulin is the main class of antibodies in tears and milk, and in the respiratory, intestinal and urogenital tracts. IgM has a critical role in defending the surface of our bodies from microorganisms."[55]

> ## Evidence suggests Reishi's ability to alleviate food sensitivities.

"Morishige also noticed that Reishi seemed to balance levels of IgG, the major class of antibodies found in blood serum.[56] Where there is inflammation on the surface of the body,[57] IgG advances to the site as the major defense against microorganisms. It coats them with an identifying marker flagging other members of the immune system to finish off the invader. A toxin-neutralizer, IgG enhances phagocytosis and is in the class of antibodies that provides the newborn with acquired immunity from the mother.[58] Whether the effects Dr. Morishige noticed can be attributed to a purely `anti-allergic' or `immunomodulating' action, or even both, is academic at this point. Taken together, these actions can be described as `adaptogenic' and certainly a *Fu Zheng* action — supporting and normalizing the healthy body functions."

"You know, Ken, IgG is responsible for most types of food sensitivities. I use several herbs that inhibit IgG to desensitize people now. I'll bet that Reishi would work also," I added.

"Is there any more to the allergy story?"

"There are a few more chemical mechanisms to go through", and off he went again, referring to his files and notes.

> ## Other anti-allergy agents in Reishi are oleic acid, sulphur and a protein.

Oleic Acid

"The anti-allergic aspect of Reishi doesn't end with the ganoderic acids but goes on to include at least three other kinds of compounds. One of these is `oleic acid,' a colourless, unsaturated fatty acid occurring as an oily liquid found in tallow and in many fatty oils, including almond and olive oil (*Olea* species), from which it takes its name.

"Oleic acid was isolated as an active constituent of Reishi mycelium by the Japanese in 1987. They determined that this common acid significantly inhibits the release of histamine from rat mast-cells and in a dose-dependant manner; the more oleic acid, the more inhibition. Although oleic acid slightly decreased mast-cell content of cyclic AMP, it still inhibited histamine release, in part by stabilizing cell membranes."[59]

Sulphur

"In continued efforts to discern the secret of Reishi's reputation in the treatment of chronic bronchitis, the same team uncovered a form of sulphur as an anti-allergic constituent of the mycelium called `cyclooctasulphur.' The mechanism of its action was not clear. Contents of cyclic AMP were not affected, but cyclooctasulphur very strongly inhibited histamine release from mast cells."[37]

Ling Zhi-8

"An immunomodulating protein from the mycelium named `Ling Zhi-8' (LZ-8) has certain anti-allergic actions too, but like the sulphur constituent, how it works isn't entirely clear. LZ-8 occurs in very small amounts in the mycelium and was isolated in Japan in 1988. Its contribution to the activity of the whole fungus as used in folk and popular medicine isn't clear at this time either, nor whether it occurs in the fruit body at all, although that is very likely.[60]

"Experiments in animals found that LZ-8 significantly reduces but doesn't entirely shut down antibody production, and that it is active in preventing severe Type I hypersensitivity reactions. Mice receiving injections of the protein two times a week displayed none of the symptoms that mice without LZ-8 had when administered an i.v. injection of a powerful allergen. The mice without LZ-8 had convulsions, rapid breathing, and death from anaphylactic shock. The mice pretreated with LZ-8 didn't have anaphylactic reactions. LZ-8 also prevented the development of autoimmune diabetes (Type I)[60] from developing in mice, indicating that it may be useful in other kinds of type IV hypersensitivity reactions such as contact dermatitis and ulcerative colitis."

Once again we had hit pay dirt. I'd already been using Reishi in the clinic for immune function problems, cancer and for cardiovascular problems. These three areas dominated any health practitioner's caseload. Now it was clear that another major health condition was responding positively to Reishi.

Over the next couple of months I started using Reishi for allergies, and to my delight it was fairly successful, especially in the case of respiratory allergies.

One of the applications I was most interested in was allergies related to *Candida albicans* infestation. This fungus type syndrome was unfortunately almost pandemic. *Candida* increases the levels of other allergies in more severe cases. The problem, I feared, was that *Candida*-related syndrome patients had to avoid mushrooms.

There seemed to be some evidence that, unlike other mushrooms, both Shiitake and Reishi would not make the *Candida* worse. True to form, not only did the *Candida* patients not get worse, but they responded very favorably to Reishi. The allergies almost immediately subsided and their *Candida* index (an indicator of the seriousness of the problem) dropped faster than with regular therapies.

I was certainly starting to view Reishi as a major tool in my clinical practice. It helps patients deal with some of the five major areas I see in the clinic. This meant that I was using Reishi with almost 40% of my patients. I was starting to gather a large amount of personal experience with this special herb as well.

I kept coming back to the same central phenomenon: Reishi calms people. The calming effect alleviates most of their problems. Reishi seemed to have effects as "advertised." It affected the immune system and influenced cardiovascular problems and allergic reactions. But the calming, almost contented feeling it seems to deliver to the patient was a central theme.

In a high stress modern world, this is probably the most important benefit I can give many of my patients.

Chapter 6

Exploring Other Health Effects
of Reishi

Ken, we have looked at many areas with this herb, but we have yet to look at the key area of longevity. This is the phenomenon that is at the center of many of the myths related to Reishi. We should look into it a little more deeply."

When I returned to wrap up our discussion, we explored the areas of longevity, liver protection, neuromuscular disorders, diabetes and altitude sickness.

Anti-Aging

> Reishi works as an anti-oxidant against free radicals, protects against the effects of radiation and has anti-inflammatory effects.

"The next thing I looked at was the idea of longevity. I found information on the role of anti-oxidants against 'free radical' chemicals in the body, Reishi's ability to counteract the effects of radiation and more data on its anti-inflammatory attributes," Ken continued.

" As most people are now aware, the infamous 'free radical electron' is the subject of numerous articles in the popular health press and the scientific literature on aging. The free radical continues to be of intrinsic concern in the prevention of disease and the preservation of youth.

" An oxygen molecule with an unpaired or 'free' electron is created as part of the immune response in the destruction of unwanted cells such

81

as tumors and viruses, and in formidable quantities by X-rays in the radiotherapy of cancer. Like too much radiation, the free radicals from sunlight can cause cancer by damaging cellular DNA. Free radicals can also cause our tissues to become brittle and our skin to wrinkle, mutate our DNA, cause our blood to clot abnormally, alter connective tissue, disrupt lubricants in our joints, and constricted capillaries and small arteries.[18]

"The gradual depletion of the body's free radical protectants as we age is part of the `free radical theory' of aging. Supplementation of free radical protectants is the subject of advances in preventative medicine.[18] Besides various amino acids, *Beta*-carotene, vitamins C, E, B-1, B-6, zinc and selenium, certain bioflavonoids in herbs, fruits and vegetables act as free radical `scavengers,' pairing the unpaired oxygen radicals and rendering them harmless.

"Free radical-caused degeneration at the cellular level is considered by many to be the most important factor in the process of aging.

"At the Beijing College of Traditional Chinese Medicine in 1985, Wang Jifeng and co-workers used free radical systems to see what effect, if any, Reishi might have in scavenging the two most destructive free radicals known, superoxide and the hydroxyl radical. Their purpose was to explore the validity of Reishi's traditional reputation as an aging-retardant from the perspective of free radical scavenging."[20]

> ## Free radicals decrease by 50% with the use of Reishi.

"An earlier study of Reishi by the same team found the fungus improved the function of red blood cells in transferring oxygen, an apparently intrinsic part of Reishi's therapeutic action in the treatment of disease and the improvement of health. They add that there is a relationship here to the adenosine abundant in Reishi, but that adenosine is not a free radical scavenger.[20]

"What they wanted to know was whether the fungus was detoxifying or scavenging the oxygen at the same time it was improving the flow, for too much oxygen can lead to free radical formation. By analyzing the blood plasma of rabbits previously injected with Reishi (0.48g/kg x 2/ day x 2.5), they were able to determine that the natural scavenging activity of blood plasma on hydroxyl radicals was significantly enhanced. (Free radical scavenging, as indicated by a 50.4% drop in ethylene production, was significantly enhanced by Reishi.)[20]

"In other types of experiments, Reishi scavenged the superoxide radical at a significant rate. The more Reishi, the higher the rate of scavenging. And if Reishi was given constantly, the action was a lasting one.[20] This indicates that for best results Reishi should betaken according to a regular daily schedule.

"Exactly what the antioxidants are in Reishi was not determined.[20] It may be that like some other anti-aging herbs in Chinese medicine, Reishi acts through another route — potentiating or stimulating the body's own free radical scavenger, an enzyme called 'superoxide dismutase,' or for short, SOD."[21] *

"You mean they left the work there?" I interrupted.

"No. Important findings were to follow," Ken replied. "But first, let's look back in time, way back," he added.

"The ancients noted another type of Reishi they called the purple fungus or *Zi zhi* (*Ganoderma japonicum* or *G. sinense* Zhao, Xu and Zhang).[17] Today this same fungus is commonly sold in the markets of China and Japan and, like the red fungus we know as Reishi or *Ling zhi*, it was said to increase the life-span. However, this one was also used to strengthen the spirit, treat deafness, improve the complexion and relieve afflictions of the joints. It seems this mushroom was also applied to circulation and heart conditions, for the ancients used it to cure lack of work energy and stamina, painful chest, bad nerves and abnormal coldness of the feet." refer to Chapter 1 Notes, *Ben Coa*

"In any case, I suspect the scientists investigating Reishi for anti-aging effects took their clue for free radical scavenging properties from the part about improving the complexion and relieving afflictions of the joints."

> ## Reishi protects against cobalt X-ray radiation.

"The polysaccharides of *Zi zhi* were studied at the Institute of Industrial Hygiene in Jiangxi Province in China," continued Ken, "to determine their protective effect on bone marrow cells exposed to cobalt X-ray radiation. The polysaccharides produced a radioprotective effect comparable to that provided by the amino acid L-cysteine,[17] an especially active scavenger of free radical electrons.

---

* At the Department of Biology at Peking University in Beijing, Yao-Ren Dai and colleagues found the alternative route (free radical scavenging by SOD potentiation) in several medicinal plants from traditional Chinese medicine as they investigated an herbal role in 'delaying the aging process.' Experiments with mice fed various herbal extracts showed that an extract of Hawthorn berries (*Crataegus pinnatifida*) produced the strongest statistically significant rates of SOD activity stimulation — by approximately 137% in female mice and 109% in males, compared to mice without the extract.

" A more dramatic demonstration of Reishi's radioprotective action was carried out by Chinese scientists who subjected mice to sufficient levels of cobalt 60 to induce `acute radiation sickness.' Although eventually all the mice died from the exposure, an injection of Reishi following a lethal dose of radiation caused a marked prolongation of their survival time. Administered (intra-gastrically) before and after the lethal dose of radiation however, Reishi produced an impressive preventive effect. Given 20 days prior to irradiation and continued for 14 days after, Reishi caused a significant reduction in the death rate.[1]

"Since the liver is one of the organs that is most likely to age quickly, I turned to that subject next," Ken commented.

Liver Protection

> ## Alcohol extract of Reishi aids against liver necrosis and hepatitis.

"There are impressive reports from China and Japan of Reishi's beneficial effects on the liver.[1,22,23] From all indications so far, however, a raw product or a water extract form will have little or no effect, whereas an alcoholic or other type of solvent extract of Reishi possesses significant effects.

A Korean study in 1987 determined that the concurrent administration of Reishi extract (200 mg/kg) with the free radical scavenging amino acid glutathione (100 mg/kg) reduced the damage to liver cells and changes in fatty acid deposits of rat livers more than either could alone. These substances combined (100 plus 100 mg/kg), in a pretreatment of rats subjected to a powerful liver damaging agent (carbon tetrachloride), provided a significant degree of liver protection. The results indicated that the combination is particularly beneficial against liver necrosis and hepatitis."[24]

"It is easy to see that Reishi doesn't increase the longevity of the rat. The number of rats that have been sacrificed for Reishi research must be in the hundreds by now," I joked.

"Try thousands," Ken added.

" A more humane liver injury model for testing drugs and herbs was developed recently in Japan. Using cultured rat liver cells, a comparison was made of the liver cell protection action of a Reishi fruit body extract to that of a Reishi mycelial extract and two other natural products, glycyrrhetinic acid, (a known liver protectant derived from licorice root), and an extract of *Alismatis rhizoma*.[25]

"Against the chemically-induced liver cell damage in this model, the only product to provide a significant level of prevention was the Reishi fruit body extract.[25] However so, a freeze-dried mycelial product was tested in Japan in liver failure patients with good results. Taking a rather large dose of 50 grams dissolved in water (300 ml) 3 times daily for a period of six months, blood measurements showed the Reishi mycelium has a `significant therapeutic effect.'[22]

"This was clearly evident in a dramatic drop of serum levels of body chemicals measured to determine liver intoxication (serum glutamate-pyruvate transaminase (GPT) and glutamine-oxaloacetic acid transaminase (GOT), which fell, in one example, from 450 to 85 IU/1 GPT and from 270 to 65 IU/1 GOT.[22]

"Studies in Beijing discovered that alcoholic extracts, whether of Reishi or *Zi zhi*, repeatedly demonstrated liver-protectant activity by decreasing liver accumulation of fatty acid (triglyceride) as well as lowering levels of GPT in the serum of liver-damaged mice.[26,27] And yes, as you may have surmised, Terry, there is a connection here to Reishi and the heart.

"While triglyceride levels in the liver are an indication of liver damage or disease, blood levels of triglycerides are measured as an indication of predisposition to coronary heart disease. Then again, there are people with normal amounts of triglycerides in their blood who have dangerously high levels of serum cholesterol and the reverse situation can be found too."

Reishi lowers triglycerides in 68 - 74% of patients at risk for heart diseases.

"Triglyceride readings, though not a reliable indicator of heart disease risk, are taken anyway because they are still closely tied to high levels of cholesterol. By lowering triglyceride levels, cholesterol counts are more likely to drop at the same time, but again, not always.

"In one study, Reishi was found effective in lowering triglyceride levels in 68% of coronary heart disease patients[28] and in another study in 74.4% of hyperlipidemic patients.[29] Oddly enough, two other trials found Reishi increased triglyceride levels. In 72 hyperlipidemic patients, triglyceride levels increased in 14% while decreasing in 52%![30] This incongruent finding is, I suspect, due to the liver adjusting to eliminating and processing more fats than it could previously.

"In patients with high blood pressure, after three months on Reishi, mean levels of triglycerides had increased, though not significantly (138.7 to 150.7 mg/dl). After another three months the mean level dropped to below levels at the beginning of the trial (138.7% to 133.7 mg/dl), though again, not by a significant amount. Total cholesterol, on the other hand, was significantly reduced by the end of the six month trial.[31]

"At the Department of Pharmacology at the Institute of Materia Medica in Beijing, Liu Geng-tao and coworkers provided even more dramatic evidence of *Ganoderma's* liver-protectant action when they administered extracts to mice in which the greater part of their livers were surgically removed. In the form of alcoholic extracts, Reishi and *Zi zhi* `promoted regeneration' of the livers.[26]

"The same experiment was repeated to compare various solvent preparations of Reishi mycelium and spores."

Reishi helps to regenerate the liver.

"In a very high dose (20 g/kg), an alcohol-water soluble extract of dried mycelium (*Ganoderma capense*, a red Reishi) significantly protected mice from death induced by a lethal dose of the anti-inflammatory drug indomethacin. In high amounts, indomethacin induces gastrointestinal tract ulcers and holes which lead to death. Not a single animal died on the mycelial extract, while 9 out of 10 of those without it perished.[23]

"The researchers concluded that the mycelial extracts probably accelerated the rate at which the liver transforms the toxin and its subsequent bile excretion.[23] In high doses and to some degree in normal doses, *Ganoderma* may be classified as a liver detoxicant and protectant. In traditional Chinese medicine, Reishi is prescribed for the treatment of mushroom poisoning (120 grams simmered in water) and chronic hepatitis.[32]

"Reishi appears to accelerate the clearance of drugs from the system through its effect on the liver. For example, instead of prolonging the anesthesia of hexobarbital, it actually shortened the time mice slept following an injection of the anesthetic.[33] This is quite the opposite of what one would anticipate from something regarded as a mild sedative and experimentally shown to elicit a caffeine-antagonizing and a muscle relaxant action, attributed to depressing or calming the central nervous system. These actions would help to explain Reishi's folk-use for people who have a difficult time getting to sleep.

Insomnia relieved by Reishi.

"Long regarded as a treatment for insomnia, *Ganoderma* significantly elevated (6.5%) the amount of slow wave sleep in rats after they drank a water extract of the fruit body for 7 days (10 grams thrice boiled in 800 ml water). No one knows why just yet, but during the week of withdrawal, when the rats had only plain water to drink, slow wave sleep at night increased even more, to 11.1%."[34]

"That is interesting because I have been using Reishi for insomnia quite successfully. It is also interesting that some Oriental theories have liver metabolism problems at the core of certain types of insomnia," I added.

"In the treatment of chronic hepatitis," Ken continued, "one recipe calls for the fruit body to be dried and then ground to powder before taking it in hot water (boiled) in a dose of 1.5 grams, 3 times daily.[32] A Reishi syrup consisting of an alcoholic extract with 10% fruit body is also prescribed for hepatitis in China, 20 ml to be taken 2 times a day, initially for a period of 30 to 90 days. One survey found Reishi effective in 70.7 to 98% of hepatitis patients treated for from 15 to 106 days. However, best results are reported in cases where the function of the liver is less severely impaired.[1]

"Only a few of the active constituents are known. In Tokyo, researchers isolated two `strongly anti-hepatotoxic' ganoderic acids from the mycelium of Reishi, namely ganoderic acids R and S.[35] Along with these, one more from the mycelium was identified, ganoderic acid T, plus a steroidal constituent named `ganodosterone,' a liver function stimulant and liver protectant. The latter is now formulated in Japan into a tablet consisting of 50 mg ganodosterone and 950 mg lactose.[36]

"These constituents occur only in small amounts. For example, it would take 10 kilograms of mycelium to yield the 50 mg needed to make one tablet. Ganoderic acids R, S and T occur in still smaller amounts.[36] S is also one of the least active of the 8 anti-hypertensive ganoderic acids isolated from the fruit body, while R, S and T so far appear to be the major triterpenoids of the mycelium."

"What have we been seeing when it comes to the neurological level?" I asked.

"Well, again I can say that there is a fair amount of material," Ken replied.

Calming effects on the nervous system are noted after consumption of Reishi.

Neuromuscular Disorders

"In China, Reishi is commonly used for neurasthenia. Neurasthenia is a neurosis with lassitude or tiredness, or neurotic debility affecting various parts of the body. It often accompanies depression where it will typically be experienced as a sensation of pressure on the larynx and a dull constriction or pressure on the lobes of the brain.

"Accordingly, Reishi is prescribed to patients who have debility following a prolonged illness, and to anorexics and insomniacs.[1] I must confess that I had hoped to cover these applications in greater detail, but the events in China in June of 1989 prevented me from getting any more information. Perhaps in the future I'll be able to tell you more."

Stress-induced tension, myasthenia gravis and muscular dystrophy have all been treated with Reishi with varying degrees of success.

"In Japan, studies of Reishi in the treatment of patients with environmental stress-induced mental diseases are preliminary at this time, but I can tell you the results are promising. In high doses (50grams 3 times daily in hot water), a ten-month study found the administration of the mycelium as a food-additive to patients suffering from psychological stresses was therapeutically significant,[3] as it was in Alzheimer's disease in patients observed for a period of eight months on Reishi mycelium.[4]

"Physicians in China found noticeable improvements in muscular dystrophy patients taking *Ganoderma*.[7-13]

"In 1974, the Department of Neurology at the Beijing Friendship Hospital began administering spore preparations of Reishi to patients with myotonia dystrophica, a rare hereditary disease related to muscular dystrophy that progresses slowly to include cataracts, atrophy of the pituitary, gonads, adrenal glands, thyroid and parathyroid, and the muscles. Atrophy of the muscles commonly begins with the face and then moves on to affect the larynx and muscles of the neck. Eventually, all the muscles in the body are affected.[7]

"The hospital scientists tried a wide assortment of agents to treat this disease but to no avail. Among these were quinine, ATP, glucose-insulin infusion, prednisone, licorice root, and a number of herbal preparations from traditional medicine. Licorice root was the only exception, but unfortunately provided only occasional relief of symptoms.[7]

"After treatment with Reishi spores and discharge from the hospital, the progress of ten patients was followed for an average of just over five years. Before leaving the hospital, each patient received intramuscular injections of a water soluble spore preparation in a daily dose of 400 mg ranging from 96 to 450 days of treatment. In addition, three patients received powdered Licorice root in combination with the spore injections for one to two months.[7]

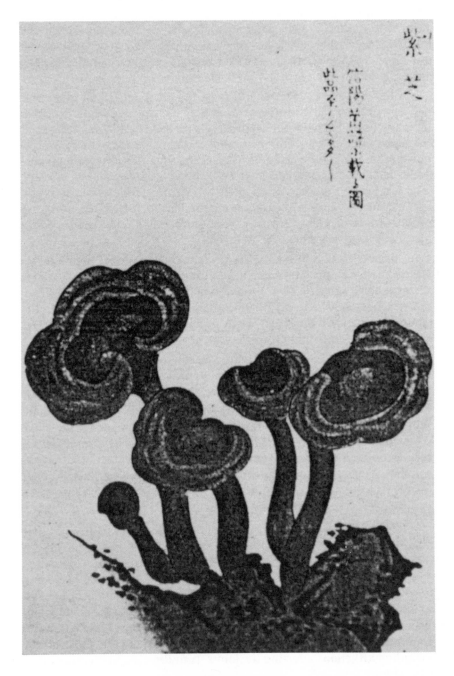

An Old Depiction of Reishi
from the Japanese book *Ben Cao Tu Pu.* (repro: Hadeler)

"In 1982, the hospital reported that the patients had started to show benefits back in 1974, after their first 7 to 14 days of treatment. The first signs of improvement were seen in physical strength, sleep and appetite. Then came relief of general symptoms and weight gain. When the injections were stopped, five of the ten patients had greatly improved muscle strength and their general symptoms were either completely gone or only partially remained.[7]

"Before therapy two patients were unable to raise their heads but had no problem doing so afterward. Before the spore injections, eight of the patients had problems chewing their food, but following treatment the same patients who would have taken over an hour to finish a meal now accomplished the task in a quarter the time. There were improvements in slurred speech and in one case no fatigue after an hour's walk, whereas before the treatment a mere ten minute stroll would bring on fatigue. These were the short-term results. The long-term benefits were more evident in milder cases in younger patients who had a shorter history of the disease to begin with.[7]

"In one case, a boy 13 years of age whose muscles were clearly wasting away, showed the benefits of the injections he received (96 days) six years later when he evidenced almost normal muscle strength. Two other teenage boys, 17 and 19, who were moderately afflicted with the disease to begin with, kept up their improvement over five years later and could handle doing light physical work.[7]

"In another four patients, which were severe cases, three of whom were also elderly, the results were poor in the long-term. Yet, for another three it appeared the disease had ceased to progress. The authors neglected to mention which patients received the licorice powder, but I think the results speak for themselves."

"What was it Dr. Wu said the ancients used *Ganoderma* for?" I asked. "Something about work energy and nerves, wasn't it?"

"Yes," Ken replied. And then to refresh our memory he pulled out the file on folklore again. The parallels unfolded before us like a case of `whodunit.'

"Here it is," Ken went on, "the very thing to try for neuromuscular disorders would be *Zi zhi*, the purple-black Reishi, or the *Chi zhi*, the red Reishi. Both mushrooms were said by the ancients to be useful in treating chest pains — to increase the life-span and to keep the body agile (*Chi zhi*), or to have a positive effect on the `limberness of the body' (*Zi zhi*). And while *Chi zhi* was prescribed to increase the `intellectual capacity' and `banish forgetfulness,' *Zi zhi* was a cure for lack of work energy and stamina and was believed to `strengthen the *ch'i* related to those areas,' including afflictions affecting the joints. (See *Ben Cao*, Further Readings Chp.1)

"Now, neurologically speaking, *Zi zhi* was used in treatments of fretful nerves, obscured eyesight, listlessness and deafness, and was indicated for patients who had completely lost the desire to drink or eat, or when 'the mouth cannot operate properly for speech.' For some reason this old pharmacopoeia states the fungus was also regarded as a sure cure for piles. But as we can see from the recent application in myotonia dystrophica, the effects the ancients observed thousands of years ago are a perfect match for this disease. (see also *Ben Cao*)

"Promising effects in neurological disease, muscular dystrophy and myotonia dystrophica with the spores and mycelium led to animal studies to isolate the active components involved. Tests with injections of water extracts of *Zi zhi* mycelium (20 mg/kg) were conducted by the Institute of Materia Medica of the Chinese Academy of Medical Sciences in Beijing.[8]

"This led to the isolation of two active constituents: uridine, one of the four nucleosides found in RNA, and uracil from the mycelium of a red fungus called *Bao Gai Ling Zhi* (*G. capense*). Along with a saponin peculiar to soybeans (soyasapogenol B),[11] adenosine showed up in the mycelium too. Uridine was previously applied in a very rare form of anemia with excellent results.[14] As uridine triphosphate, there are European claims of its value in treating muscle weakness and muscular atrophy.[15]

"I have two other areas of interest. Then we can call it a day," Ken said.

The Question of Diabetes

> Reishi helps moderate the physiology of diabetics.

"Reishi's use in the treatment of insomnia, gastric ulcers, liver disorders, chronic hepatitis, neurasthenia, arthritis, nephritis, asthma, bronchitis, hypertension and poisoning is part of its traditional Oriental application. Its use in treating diabetes is much less recognized and at the outset one would tend to think Reishi was not appropriate for this affliction. A clinical study in China with heart disease and chronic bronchitis patients found blood glucose 'markedly increased.'[1]

"However, there are undeniable reports of blood sugar reduction or 'hypoglycemic' action recognized from clinical experience in Chinese and Japanese applications. These are corroborated in animal experiments.[61-64]

"Acknowledging that some believe Reishi to be efficacious in this disease, Dr. Morishige couldn't say one way or the other about Reishi's success, in spite of the fact that he sees numerous diabetics and has attempted to treat them with Reishi.

"He explains that the majority of these diabetics opt for insulin treatment alone because it is commonly recognized in Japan that insulin is considerably more effective. Another reason is that the diabetic tends to abhor the bitter taste associated with drinking Reishi preparations. Because of these factors, Dr. Morishige has not had sufficient data to arrive at any conclusions as to its efficacy in diabetes.[52]

"If animal studies are any indication, and usually they are, then there is something to this use after all. As to the belief that Reishi might cure diabetes, that remains to be proven in humans. Nonetheless, diabetics using Reishi for whatever reason would be wise to monitor changes in their blood sugar. Animal studies indicate they may find that they need less insulin.

"Studies by the Asahi Chemical Industry Co., Ltd. of Osaka, Japan, found that rats with experimentally-induced diabetes, fed on a large dose (1 gram/kg) of powdered Reishi mycelium in the form of a water suspension, had a dramatic decrease in their blood sugar. It took only six hours for it to drop from approximately 425 mg/dl to 350 mg/dl.[64]

"Renowned medicinal plant pharmacologist Hiroshi Hikino had earlier conducted his own investigations of this activity in mice. He used a water extract of the fruit body prepared by boiling Reishi (1 kg/10 l water) for two hours at 95°C until the water reduced in volume to a tenth the amount. In normal mice a large dose (the equivalent of 10 g fruit body/kg) produced a significant degree of hypoglycemic activity. A drop in blood glucose of 31% was registered, even a day later. Two polysaccharides (*Beta*-D-glucans) were isolated as the active constituents and named ganoderans A and B.[61]

"In mice with experimentally induced diabetes, doses of 10, 30 and 100 mg/kg produced significant results, with ganoderan A showing more activity than ganoderan B. With A (10 mg/kg), after 7 hours there was a significant drop in blood glucose of 43%, while with the same dose of B the drop (11%) was barely significant.[61]

"The following year, Hikino joined Masashi Tomoda and others at the Kyoritsu College of Pharmacy in Tokyo to examine a sample of Reishi from Kyoto. This time, ganoderan B turned up, but not A. Instead, they found another ganoderan with hypoglycemic activity which they named ganoderan C, a somewhat less active polysaccharide than ganoderan B.[62]

"This demonstrates once again that with plants from one growing area to the next and with fungi from one growing area and one strain to the next, there are going to be variations and at times differences in the occurrence of active constituents.

"Other studies of Reishi's potential anti-diabetic properties have shown that in high doses a water extract of the fruit body is effective by the oral route in 200 to 1000 mg/kg doses,[63,64] which translates to roughly 17 grams of Reishi for an adult human, assuming equivalency will apply.

"In animals with an experimentally-induced increase in levels of blood glucose and inhibited insulin secretion from the pancreas, the water extract of Reishi prevented not only the blood glucose increase but did so without affecting the level of insulin in the blood.[63]

"A similar test was performed using orally administered glucose. Ten minutes after the glucose, Reishi reduced the increase of insulin caused by the glucose and reduced the increase of glucose in plasma. And when insulin levels in the untreated rats were dropping, plasma levels of insulin in the Reishi-treated rats maintained their high level. The mechanism of this seemingly protective action on insulin levels is an excellent candidate for future investigation."[63]

An Altitude Adaptogen

"In keeping with Reishi's ancient reputation as a rejuvenating supplement of mountain-dwelling ascetics, here's an interesting fact. Workers from China requisitioned to the highlands of Tibet are provided with *Ganoderma tablets* to reduce the effects of altitude sickness."

> Reishi oxygenates the blood to alleviate elevation sickness.

"One of the principle roles of Reishi is that of an oxygenator. A marked increase in blood oxygen was noticed from clinical studies of patients with pulmonary heart disease and chronic bronchitis treated with a Reishi syrup.[1] Also, in animal studies, a solution of Reishi mycelium enhanced hypoxia endurance.[65] Hypoxia is a reduced supply of oxygen to the tissues — less than normal levels — regardless of an adequate supply from the blood.

"The supply of oxygen is much lower at high altitudes. The `thinner air' causes people who have travelled from a low altitude to a high one to commonly experience `unadapted symptoms,' which for some people can be extreme. Among these symptoms are breathlessness, headaches, dizziness, insomnia, palpitation and vomiting. When these symptoms occur together the diagnosis is something called `acute plateau un-adapted syndrome.'[65]

"Based on the increased endurance to hypoxia found in animals given Reishi, researchers at the Hunan Institute of Pharmaceutical Industry decided to test an extract in people who work at high altitudes. Made into a tablet, the Reishi mycelial extract either alleviated or reduced unadapted symptoms in 17 of 19 persons.[65]

"This early success led to tests in a much larger number of people and included a comparison of two different preparations. *Number One* preparation was a tabletted extract of the liquid mycelia and *Number Two*, a tabletted extract of the fruit body. Candidates were selected after they had entered high elevations in Tibet and Qinghai. Only those without complicated reactions or tendency to car sickness were included.[65]

"Subjects took 3 tablets twice daily, 6 days in a row, while travelling in covered trucks in severe cold. They started at an elevation of 3700 meters and after 6 days had reached an elevation of 4750 meters. Of 900 subjects on the No. 1 tablet, 94.1% experienced no vomiting and 82.4% no headache.[65]

"The results with No. 2 tablet were not substantially different. Of 976 subjects, 83.7% had no headaches and 96.1% experienced no vomiting. Similar results were seen in 225 subjects using the No. 1 tablet, who showed an overall 98.6% rate of prevention or no symptoms, and in 244 subjects on No. 2 tablets who showed a 97.5% rate of prevention. There were no signs of toxicity or side-effects in any of the tests conducted.[65]

"Compared to a tally of acute unadapted symptoms made by the Academy of Army Medicine, which showed between 77.2 and 83% of subjects without some form of medication experience symptoms, the 16.2 to 27.8% of those on Reishi who had any unadapted symptoms in a series of tests clearly indicates the mushroom has definite advantages for people travelling to high altitudes.[65]

"Well that about wraps it up, Terry. We dug up a fair amount of material on Reishi. Imagine what we'd have if we could read Japanese and Chinese characters. It's too bad that all that untranslated research material has to be left untouched!

"In any event, Terry, the amount of material on Reishi that we've collected on its immune system effects, cancer, heart-related problems and so on, could fill a filing cabinet."

And that was my last marathon meeting with Ken.

I now had more information to expand the range of problems I could prescribe Reishi for. Reishi works on longevity as an antioxidant, squelching free radicals — one of the most important factors in aging. It has also been shown that Reishi can protect the human body from X-ray radiation, an important fact, especially for cancer patients undergoing radiation therapy.

The protective properties for the liver also added support to Reishi's reputation as a longevity herb. I wasn't a bit surprised about the research related to insomnia or calming of the central nervous system, as I had been using it clinically for these problems for months now.

I was certainly going to add Reishi to programs I directed for many diabetics. I had some familiarity with high elevation sickness as several mountain climbers were patients, including some members of the Canadian Mount Everest climbing team. I was eager to pass on this information to them.

I must admit though, I was starting to feel like a Reishi evangelist. Was I the only person in North America using Reishi so intensely? I decided that my next stage of research was to interview several prominent figures in the North American herbal community, both practitioners and those in the herb industry.

What would their response be to my questions about Reishi? So far, the purpose of the research had been to gather information for my own clinical use. The next stage was to integrate this information with the knowledge of modern practitioners and manufacturers.

Chapter 7

Reishi in the Clinic

After many months of travel and research, the focus of my activities turned to speaking to health practitioners who were familiar with Reishi. I wanted to ask the most experienced practitioners and commentators in North America how they used Reishi and what results they achieved.

The Clinic by the Bay

San Anselmo stands as a small island of calm in the bustle of San Francisco's Bay Area communities. Nestled at the foot of Mount Tamalpais, uphill from San Rafael on the peninsula north of San Francisco itself, San Anselmo's core is a pleasant set of town buildings and well kept boutiques and stores.

Just a few footsteps from this picturesque setting is a quiet side street. The day I visited, it was a sunny mild July afternoon and pleasant just to walk the shady sidewalks. A small building with a flat front was my goal. From a distance it was neat in appearance but otherwise unremarkable. At close range the building's uniqueness became clear. In the windows were large glass jars full of dark liquid and floating objects — more roots, herbs and what looked suspiciously like a lizard or two!

A pair of beautiful ornate wooden doors opened under a sign *Pine Street Chinese Benevolent Association*. As a traveller to Chinatowns all over the world, this Benevolent Association seemed a bit out of place but one could hardly ask for a nicer setting.

Through the doors the smells and sounds were more familiar. I was greeted by a large room with a tall ceiling perhaps 15 feet high. On the left was a long large mahogany counter and behind it the wall of wooden boxes which spell one thing: Oriental herb store. Something was different however. There were no posters for products, no glittering plastic packages. No chatter of bartering customers and staff. To the right of the doors an elegant artificial fountain gurgled and sputtered. It was made of some sort of metal, perhaps copper, and cast a calming effect on the high-ceiling room. Bookcases and comfortable couches lined the wall.

Behind the counter, people who looked like apprentices were collecting herbal materials and combining them into formulas and packaging them (as is traditional) in paper containers, folded like sturdy origami. Customers came and went in regular succession.

I had come to San Anselmo to meet Michael Broffman, an American who had studied Chinese medicine and art in Taiwan many years before such interests were common. Michael was known to me by reputation. He had worked hard to support a system of training acupuncturists in California through apprenticeship. Typically, C.A.'s (Certified Acupuncturists) are trained for four years in accredited schools throughout the state. Michael had convinced the state bureaucrats that students could be legitimately and thoroughly trained in the old manner, teacher to student. It was an approach I respected deeply since I had some experience with it while working with the Indians of Alberta and British Columbia.

Michael had added a profoundly modern aspect to the Pine Street dispensary. With the help of a retired engineer and an industrious apprentice, Michael had encouraged the development of a system to reproduce the human pulse on the screen of a computer and then analyze it according to traditional Oriental medical theory. It was an exciting project.

For years I've been using various techniques for examining the state of individual health. The Oriental pulse system is extremely effective but requires an intimidating amount of skill and practice to use. Michael's project promised at least the hope of accelerated learning.

A rustling from the back of the large room indicated the end of a client's appointment. A long hallway extended back into the building and there were tantalizing peeks of other offices or examining rooms. In a moment, Michael appeared. He's a vital man, perhaps forty though his appearance speaks more of thirty. A bit shorter than my height, 5' 8", he had the slimness and vigour of an athlete. Clean-shaven, with his black-brown hair slightly long at the back, he portrayed the very image of competence and vitality with a touch of mystery thrown in.

After a few minutes of introductions and greetings, Michael took me back into the office area of the Pine Street building for Chinese tea and conversation. He introduced me to Michael McCullough, the apprentice whose work on the pulse reading apparatus was so promising.

On that pleasant July afternoon we talked of many things, and sure enough an old friend was to reappear.

"What do you know about *Ling zhi*?" I said. "It's quickly becoming a popular item in health food stores but the Oriental history is much more profound."

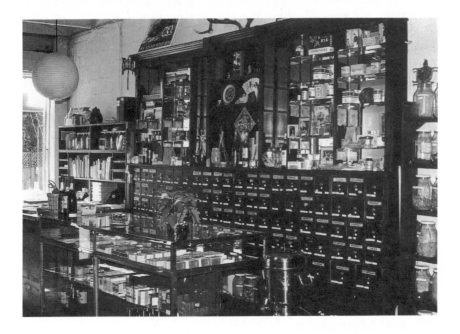

The Pine Street Clinic

A smile split Michael Broffman's face. "It is the most expensive ingredient in those jars you see in our window. Each year we create tinctures using the sun. We put precious herbal or medicinal items in rice wine, place them just right so they get a few hours of direct sunlight in the early morning . . . and wait. After several months, we have tonics and tinctures of great usefulness. *Ganoderma* is a key ingredient."

"I'm really interested in *Ling zhi*. I would be very interested to hear any stories you have about it," I added.

"I first became introduced to *Ling chih* while in the Republic of China in 1975," Michael began.

"In Chinese medicine, as you are familiar, there are several historical traditions which govern how herbs are used:

"First there is the orthodox or government view which comprises the herbal repertoire as promulgated by the current dynasty regime. The most familiar is now that passed on by the *Pen T'sao*.

"Second there is the provincial tradition. This comprises very local or regional medicine. Products are largely wildcrafted and sold fresh. They are mostly used and known by local people. Taiwan has one of the most sophisticated local medicine repertoires.

"Finally, there are the philosophical medical perspectives, with different schools using herbs in different ways for different therapeutic intentions. For example, Buddhist herbal schools of thought . . . or Tao . . . or Neo-Taoist or Neo-anything . . . Confucius, Yin-Yang School, Naturalist school and dozens more. . ."

"So that is why you can find so many different and even conflicting pieces of information on each herb?" I asked.

"Yes, and my point of view with *Ling zhi* is the very regional Confucian usage that is found in Southern Taiwan — near *Tai Dong*, a small town on the southeast coast," Michael said.

"We grade *Ling zhi*, or as we say it *Ling-chih*, by the following criteria:

Color: The deeper the color, the better. This color must penetrate the mushroom and the pigment must be distributed evenly, even in cross-section.

Size: Large and thick mushrooms are preferred. If the mushroom has an odd shape or whimsical shape, this adds to its value.

Harvesting conditions: The conditions in a mushroom's environment are important. Soil pH, foliage and nearby trees are all examined and recorded.

Weather circumstances: The general climatic conditions (amount of rainfall, etc.) can affect quality.

Presence of insects: Insect damage or activity on the mushroom decreases its value.

Root depth: The mushroom must have good anchoring but not deep.

"*Ling-chih* has many uses and its value is determined by the formula in which it is placed. This is referred to in Chinese medicine as establishing value as a direct function of context (formula). An herb has no identifiable therapeutic value until you put it in a context with other herbs. I'll describe that usage in the terminology and concepts used by traditional Chinese medicine.

"*Ling-chih* has an affinity for dead (or relatively dead), low *qi*-emitting phenomena in the body, things that are not moving or are very slow moving. If there is stagnation/excess or accumulative toxins of this description in the body (even if barricaded in by adhesions/scar tissue from whatever causes) then the situation is appropriate for *Ling-chih*. If there are toxins that would be dangerous to cleanse through the body, then this is a good *Ling-chih* situation.

"A modern use for *Ling-chih* is in co-ordination with Western radiation or chemotherapy for cancer cases. In Chinese historical texts, *Ling-chih* was used with 8-10 hours moxabustion (burning vegetable `punk' therapy) daily producing a Chinese version of radiation therapy. This treatment continued for 6 weeks with or without Chinese herbs which exert a chemotherapeutic effect on the body like *Catharanthus roseus* or modern vincristin.

"In a typical 21 day chemotherapeutic cycle (all things being equal), a modern prescription would be:

"*Ling-chih* (5-8 days) followed by detox-clearing herbs (5-8 days). Next would be tonic herbs (5-8 days), the chemotherapy followed by symptomatic treatment as needed (1 - 3 days) and then a course of *Ling-chih*. This cycle is then repeated.

"A dosage range of fresh-dried *Ling-chih* for an adult of 130 to 180 pounds might be 3-5 tablespoons daily (or 20 - 30cc i.m. injection daily).

"We have used *Ling-chih* more extensively for 10 years since it is available to us, grown locally in the Bay area and fresh-dried. Other diseases where we use a variant of the treatment process include deep recalcitrant infections especially in the very deep lung and pelvic floor.

"The dosage is quite important because left to itself *Ling chih*, even in modest doses, tends to `sink' — to go down. It is not well directed on its own. It doesn't naturally go to certain places in the body or seek out specific channels. It is lumbering in movement and slow but persistent. In order to more highly direct it, other herbs are included. Different formulas are structured around *Ling chih* to direct it. Where medicine is being limited by amount, then direction can be done with acupuncture within the first couple of hours of ingestion. Alternatively, injections can be placed into acupuncture points. The *Shu* points on the back are preferred.

"We don't want the quantity of *Ling chih* to be excessive, beyond the body's ability to assimilate. When *Ling chih* is allowed to stagnate in the body, it is very difficult to get out. A certain amount of metabolic activity is therefore required in a patient's body, either intrinsic or induced, to avoid this problem. This problem is most often spotted when higher dosages are used or the patient is a child or older person."

"Well," I said. "You've shown me a lot more subtlety in usage than I expected. It certainly indicates the power and usefulness of Reishi in skilled hands."

Our conversation then turned to Michael's other projects and activities and our meeting continued for several hours. Some of the information on Reishi was completely new and I was thrilled. The use of Reishi seemed to be an art, an art as powerful as Reishi's healing ability. I remembered several of the scientific papers mentioning a dose-dependency. Here at the clinical level it seems to be very important. Michael had also added a lot of new information on how Reishi quality was judged by traditional medical specialists.

But what about the Western tradition of medicine? Would M.D.'s have anything to contribute on the subject of clinical Reishi use?

A Doctor Bridging Two Worlds

In a vastly different setting, Dr. Andrew Weil, a Western M.D., has written some of the most elegant and thorough accounts of the holistic approach in medicine. I had heard that he was using Reishi in his clinical practice. I called him at his clinic in Tucson, Arizona and set up an interview time.

Dr. Weil is the author of *The Natural Mind, Health & Healing, Marriage of the Sun and the Moon,* and *Chocolate to Morphine,* a series of well-written books which have done a lot to open minds about holistic medical concepts. I had heard that another, *Dr. Andrew Weil's Natural Medicine,* was due to be published in 1990. Dr. Weil was well-known to me as a member of the advisory board of *HerbalGram,* North America's most respected journal of botanical medicine, the Herb Research Foundation and the American Botanic Counsel. With a B.Sc. in Botany, he was no stranger to the pharmacological power of plants.

Dr. Weil practices in Tucson, teaches medicine at the University of Arizona Medical School and maintains a busy writing and lecturing schedule. Our phone conversation began with an obvious question.

"When did your interest in mushrooms begin, Dr. Weil?"

"I have always been interested in mushrooms, but my interest picked up in the early 70s when I took mushroom identification more seriously. My main reason for this was my interest in psychotropic and toxic mushrooms. Over time my interests broadened to the general nutritional uses of mushrooms. I have been teaching classes to both professional and amateur mushroom groups since the mid - 70s."

"I was astounded that there were no medicinal uses for mushrooms in the West. I then found a very rich tradition in the Orient. One of the main mushrooms was Reishi, so I increased my research on the subject."

"What do you find it most useful for?"

"I find it best to stimulate the immune system. Reishi is a non-toxic substance which is very useful in this area."

"How do you use it?"

"I usually use it in formula, a formula that contains Shiitake, Reishi, *Polyporus umbellatus, Poria cocos,* and *Flammulina velutipes.*

"What kind of specific problems would you use it for?"

"I have been using it for three years in cancer cases, AIDS cases, pre-AIDS conditions and for depressed immunity in general. I have recently found it very useful in cases of Chronic Fatigue Syndrome. I often use it in combination with *Astragalus* and antioxidant vitamins."

This sparked my interest. "Well, Andy," I said, "I have been using it in almost the same manner for CFS. I usually add the herbs Echinacea and Licorice. Do you see much of a future for medicinal mushrooms in treating immune system problems?"

"Yes I do," he replied, "but I feel there is a need for more Western-style research on this herb."

"There has been quite a bit of research undertaken in the Orient from a Western scientific point of view, clinical studies as well," I said.

"Well, let's hope that it encourages more research here," he continued. "I feel that the research will have to be undertaken in the U.S.A. before the use of Reishi will increase substantially in North America."

"What emphasis do you place on Reishi in your practice?" I asked.

"I consider it very important. I probably prescribe it every day in my practice and I'd have to consider it one of the major substances I work with."

"What about the other medicinal mushrooms? Do you feel that they will be used more often in the coming years?"

"Yes, but the biggest problem with these products is absorption through the GI tract. Some of the medicinal ingredients have problems being absorbed."

"Do you consider the wild variety of Reishi more useful than the cultivated one?"

Dr. Weil paused for a moment. "I think almost all of the materials available are cultivated. The most important thing is the substrate or the material the mushroom is grown on."

"How would you summarize Reishi's medicinal value?"

"I feel that it can protect the immune system function, and is a general adaptogen."

I was encouraged by my discussion with Dr. Weil. Here was a Western M.D. who was actively using Reishi in a clinical situation and finding it valuable enough to prescribe on a regular basis. There was one final person on my list who I felt would round out the North American perspective on this mushroom.

An Authority on Reishi

Many times during both research and interviewing stages a name kept popping up—Dr. Subhuti Dharmananda Ph.D. From many sources I had heard that Dr. Dharmananda was the best all around academic researcher on herbal products. I was familiar with his writing over the years. Many of his articles and books were on my own library shelves.

103

After reviewing some of his articles and an extremely well done chapter on mushroom polysaccharides that he had written, I was quite eager to interview him. Managing the interview was another matter entirely. Like virtually all the experts I had contacted, Dr. Dharmananda had an extremely busy schedule. A personal visit, even an extended phone conversation, seemed like an impossibility.

Finally, modern technology came to the rescue; this time in the form of the ubiquitous fax machine. We exchanged preliminary information and Dr. Dharmananda kindly followed up with an extended commentary on Reishi.

Dr. Dharmananda made something perfectly clear from the very beginning. He was not in favour of "hyping" a single herb. His fax stated, "I use herbs in combinations clinically (or when manufacturing for clinical use), and when I write about herbs I try to write about related species with similar properties. In this case, *Ganoderma* is just one of several dozen mushrooms with polysaccharides which in lab animals inhibits growth of implanted tumor cells. Presumably, all these mushroom polysaccharides have the same effect, though their potency undoubtedly varies.

"*Ganoderma* seems somewhat unique in the area of ganoderic acids which have effects such as treating hyperlipidemia, improving oxygen utilization etc. The same type of effects can be obtained from similar types of compounds which are found in ginseng and other popular plants from Asia."

To emphasize this in his latest book he talks about polysaccharides in eight mushrooms: *Coriolus versicolor, Ganoderma sp., Tremmela sp., Grifola sp., Poria cocos, Lentinus edodes, Cordyceps, and Armillaria mellea*. He says that both Shiitake and Reishi are presently being used on ARC/AIDS patients as well as for cancer patients. Their use in America follows initial reports of success from Japan.

The fax continued, "I've been using *Ganoderma* for about five or six years. It is frequently recommended. For example, the following formulas I've designed contain it:

"*Astra 8* (for enhancing immunity), *Astra Garlic* (for lowering lipids), *Ganoderma 18* (for general tonic purposes), *Composition Tablets* (for HIV treatment).

"Our HIV treatment programs have consistently used *Ganoderma* as a dominant herb in a treatment that involves a large number of herbs. For example, in our current base formula, *Composition-A*, it makes up 12% of the prescription. We have had very good response in treatment of HIV infection, but one can't attribute that solely to *Ganoderma* (if at all)."

Dr. Dharmananda goes on to say, "The future of *Ganoderma* depends entirely on whether or not it is heavily promoted in the health food industry. It could be the next `garlic,' `Vitamin C,' or `CoQ10.' (I put in these quotations as they are phenomena as well as actual materials.) It could also be next of many Chinese herbs, well-known to the community of people who work with Chinese herbs but rarely known outside that.

"We use a combination of *G. japonicum* (which the Chinese prefer) and *G. lucidum* (which the Japanese seem to prefer) in making herb products. The former mushroom is somewhat sweeter and softer than the latter."

Dr. Dharmananda has written some great information about polysaccharides and I highly recommend his books, *Chinese Herb Therapies for Immune Disorders* and *Pearls from the Golden Cabinet*. Reading these two books will be a powerful incentive to acquire his other books.

Closer to home there were people I knew who had used Reishi and had something to contribute to my research.

Reishi in Calgary

My next interview was with Dr. David Chu, a traditional Chinese medical doctor. Dr. Chu is someone I have known for a number of years. I had travelled with him across the country many times. His clinical experience is awesome, to say the least. He worked at the Shanghai No. 2 Medical College for many years, subsequently practising and doing research in Australia and Canada.

When I first met him, he was involved in research at the University of Calgary in the area of immunology, specializing in the T- and B- lymphocyte functions. A very vital, scholarly-looking man, he is quiet at first, but once you have gained his confidence, Dr. Chu shares a wealth of information.

Even though Dr. Chu and myself both live in Calgary, our schedules rarely coincide. Ironically, I interviewed Dr. Chu in a jet 37,000 feet above earth, flying from Toronto to Calgary. We were both members of the Canadian Expert Advisory Committee for Herbs and Botanical Preparations. Because of that background, we had both gone to Ottawa for a pharmaceutical safety conference.

I was quite keen to talk to David about Reishi as I knew he would have some very practical information.

My first question focused on the main purposes for *Ling zhi* in his clinic. His comments on Reishi's general uses are as follows:

"Reishi has a *sedative* effect and will relax the central nervous system, helping with sleeplessness, anxiety and restlessness.

"Research shows that *Ling zhi* has a strong effect on the *lifespan of white blood cells (WBC)*. It increases the strength and longevity of the cells.

In turn, it will increase both the quality and the quantity of white blood cells.

"If *Ling zhi* is used at the beginning of a cold/flu it increases the WBC to aid in the decrease of the cold/flu. In the case of cancer it is especially useful. Radiation and chemotherapy lower the WBC count. When the use of *Ling zhi* is started before the treatment and used throughout the course of these therapies, the WBC won't decrease."

David has found it very useful for *asthma, bronchitis and excessive cough.* The mechanism is unknown, but he feels it has something to do with relaxing the smooth muscles of the lungs and bronchials.

"*Ling zhi* is very good for *liver function* — especially for detoxification, prevention and protection of the liver cells. It will decrease damage of the liver cells caused by viral antigen-antibody complexes," David continued. "This makes it extremely useful for hepatitis.

"*Ling zhi* is very good for the *heart* — especially palpitation, stabilizing heart function through an unknown mechanism.

"Chinese theory indicates to us that *Ling zhi* balances the five organs, toning and sedating. This is of course the theoretical basis for *Ling zhi*'s use in longevity. It is probably one of the most important longevity herbs in Chinese theory.

"It is also quite useful for *hypothyroidism*." David has had two patients with this disease and has found *Ling zhi* to be both fast and efficient without side-effects.

I followed up his comments with further questions. "What would be the more common indication you see in your clinic that would lead you to use *Ling zhi* with a patient?"

"I use it with all of my cancer patients," he began. "It is most important in that area. *Ling zhi* can neutralize toxins secreted from cancer tissue while strengthening white blood cells and stopping some of the side-effects from radiation and chemotherapy.

"I also use it extensively for menopause, especially when anxiety is associated.

"From a Chinese point of view it is important whenever you have yin deficiency. *Ling zhi* helps yin deficiency quickly and powerfully.

"I also find it useful for hypertension. Not so much to lower the blood pressure but to stabilize it when I have already lowered it using other herbs. As you understand, I usually use it in combination with other herbs but *Ling zhi* can relieve the symptoms of high blood pressure much quicker."

"Can you describe some of the clinical cases in which you have used *Ling zhi*?" I asked.

"Certainly," he said.

"I had a woman patient who had breast cancer that was stabilized by radiation therapy. She came to me after the cancer had entered the bones. After looking at her tongue I saw that she was very toxic due to the lack of moisture and dark red colour of her tongue. After two months of taking 5 (300 mg) tablets 3 times daily, her symptoms were completely stabilized, and her tongue turned back to normal.

"In a second case, a female patient had yin deficiency of the kidney. Her symptoms included blood in the urine. Her kidney function was poor according to her tongue and the pulse. Use of *Ling zhi* reduced and then stopped blood in the urine."

"Do you ever use *Ling zhi* yourself, David?"

"Yes, Terry, if I have been under lots of stress or if my schedule is very busy, *Ling zhi* can be very useful."

"How important would you consider *Ling zhi* in your practice?"

"Oh, I would consider it quite important."

"Are there any contraindications for *Ling zhi*?"

"Throughout my practice I have found it to be a very safe herb. The only contraindication would be a strong yang deficiency and quite poor digestion."

"What would you do in these situations?"

"The best way is to balance these things out first. If this is not possible, you can use a yang tonic for the yang deficiency case or a spleen stomach tonic for the poor digestion at the same time.

"I should say that we wouldn't usually use *Ling zhi* during menstruation, because it has a cooling effect, which can cause cramps."

"How long can a person take *Ling zhi*?"

"If there is no yang deficiency, it can be used for a long time. I have used it with one patient that is 93 years old. She has taken *Ling zhi* for over 10 years in small doses. And one would say that she is in very good health. Way above normal for her age."

"You can often see *Ling zhi* being carried by Taoist monks in Chinese art. Why would this be?"

"*Ling zhi* is often found in deep rain forests and on the edge of cliffs. This means that it often is collected at great risk to the collector. This is one of the reasons for it being revered. Often the harder it is to get, the more highly valued as a medicine. Because *Ling zhi* can grow from 100 to 1000 years, often the location is known but it can't be obtained because of the danger associated. It was often only obtained as part of a great heroic act, usually to save someone's life.

"It was also revered by the Taoists because it balances the five organs and thus supports longevity. This was much sought after by the Taoists. Taoists believe that *Ling zhi* was given by the gods and was perhaps a lost treasure of the gods. To them it is considered the seed of the spirit.

"There are several stories associated with *Ling zhi*.

"The best *Ling zhi* is believed to live deep in the rain forest where it is protected by snakes and tigers.

"A classic story involving *Ling zhi* revolves around a rich lord's daughter. She fell in love with a poor farm boy. This was a disgrace for her father. He had already promised her hand to another landowner's son. The daughter refused to marry the boy she was bequeathed to. She decided to run away into the deep forest instead of marrying this boy.

"Because of the disgrace, her father sent his bodyguards after her. She still refused to return. Her father then ordered her to be killed due to the dishonour. On returning to her hiding spot the soldiers found her taking a deadly poison. They left her for dead, having completed their mission with relative ease.

"The poor farm boy found her dead and carried her to a Buddhist temple and asked if the monks could bring her back to life. Of course they told him it was impossible. After great pleading they said that if a very ancient *Ling zhi* could be obtained in less than 24 hours it could bring her back to life. There was such a *Ling zhi* in one of the caves nearby. Many had tried to obtain it. All had died trying to get it because there was both a poisonous snake and a tiger protecting it.

"After several hours of dangerous pursuit, he finally tricked both the snake and the tiger and obtained the *Ling zhi*. A small portion of it brought her back to life, of course. To avoid the rage of the family they decided to live in the forest. After consuming the rest of the *Ling zhi* they both lived for several hundred years, becoming very famous for their spiritual powers. "

The airplane continued to drone on as we flew to Calgary. David had reinforced some of the knowledge I had of the clinical applications of Reishi. As a bonus, he had also added a charming story to the lore about Reishi's medicinal and spiritual powers.

When I returned to my clinic, I decided it was time to record my own clinical experiences with Reishi. I had used the product myself and suggested it to others in my clinics in Vancouver and Calgary. I had learned a great deal about Reishi in the subsequent months.

I started using Reishi in the clinic in the late fall of 1988, applying it in earnest after doing more thorough research in the early spring of 1989.

The first area I started using it in was insomnia. Many people, especially academically minded people, have a problem sleeping. The first person I used Reishi with was a professor of political science from the University of Calgary. He would continually find himself waking at 3 o'clock in the morning, not falling back to sleep until about 6:30 a.m.

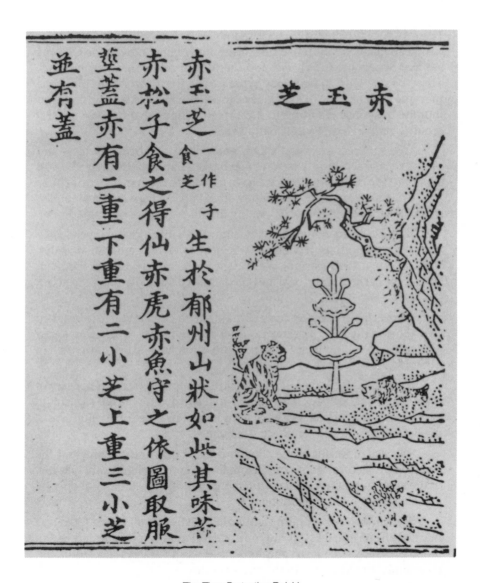

赤玉芝

赤玉芝_{食芝}一作子 生於郁州山狀如此其味苦
赤松子食之得仙赤虎赤魚守之依圖取服
蓥蓋赤有二重下重有二小芝上重三小芝
並有蓋

The Tiger Protecting Reishi
from the Ming Dynasty (1400 -) book "Tai Shang Ling Bau Zhi Cao Ping",
the first book written solely on *Ganoderma* (repro: Hadeler)

109

"This was great for getting work done during the wee hours of the morning," he said. "But now that classes are back in, I need to be rested for my morning class. It seems as though I just can't turn off my mind."

Reishi was added to his program and three weeks later, by his next visit, he was sleeping normally. After follow up visits for several months it was clear that the Reishi still worked. If he misses the Reishi for a few days, his insomnia reasserts itself. The professor noted that taking Reishi had an effect on him similar to a good meditation or even a catnap. He said he feels he will take this herb for the rest of his life.

The most common use for Reishi in my clinic now is for Chronic Fatigue Syndrome (CFS). We find that Reishi calms the person down. These people tend to be a bit "hyper." The Reishi works to build the immune system. One of the major causes of CFS is stress and lowered immune response resulting in a complete fatigue that can last several months, or in extreme cases many years.

CFS sufferers are usually very productive members of society and often exercise aerobically on a regular basis. They just lose their physical stamina. One of the problems we have noted is that when they can't be as physically active as they desire they often become very active mentally, relentlessly, even obsessively looking to find the source of their ailment.

This obsessed manner usually binds them into a vicious cycle. They have strong emotions, trying to use logic to overcome emotional issues. This, of course, is impossible. We find the Reishi calms down their system so that the cycle of emotional and physical hyperactivity ceases to strain the body.

We normally recommend 1-2 grams of powdered Reishi to be taken two times daily. The normal product for us to use is the powdered cultivated mycelium in hot water. On occasion we also use the extract in pill form.

Besides CFS, I have been using it for symptomatic relief in cases of menopause and arthritis. I also suggest Reishi during the cold season to boost immune function. We have used it in a few cases of myelofibrosis, in all cancer cases and for allergic asthma.

My use of Reishi in the clinic increased over the months that the research project was going on. Before long I noticed that Reishi was one of the most commonly used supplements in both the clinics, not only by myself, but by other practitioners.

Reishi rapidly became a standard in cardiovascular therapy. It had marked effects in at least 50% of the patients I treated for cholesterol, high blood pressure, even heart palpitations. It wasn't always successful, but it certainly added points to the success rates.

I was especially encouraged by the results found in allergies. I have seen great results in one male child eleven years old who had very bad allergic asthma. After three weeks, he was symptom free.

Food allergies also seem to respond well to treatment with Reishi. Of greatest interest to me were allergies related to *Candida albicans*, an all-too-common problem. Reishi not only lowered the rate of allergies, it decreased patient scores on the *Candida* "index." This was a little surprising since *Candida* patients often show increased symptoms when eating most mushrooms.

One of the most interesting cases is that of my accountant, Marie, who ended up with all of the signs of a healing crisis when she began to use Reishi.

A Common Western Experience

Marie LaFrange is a menopausal woman, generally in very good health, but suffering from insomnia and slight arthritis. After I became familiar with Reishi, I suggested that she take 2 tablets (300 mg. of solid extract) twice daily, to see if it would reduce her symptoms.

Within a few days Marie was complaining of aggravated symptoms and dizziness, feeling light-headed and almost drunk, an itchy scalp, increased bowel movements and especially arthritic pains. She, of course, immediately asked me what was happening. I gave a little chuckle and walked into my office. I brought back an article I had just written for a magazine. I told her to read the section on initial side effects of Reishi consumption. After she read it she realized that she had most of the symptoms. Her dosage was lowered to one tablet daily for a few days. After two days, she raised it to one tablet, twice daily and in another couple of days she was back to the original two tablets, twice daily.

Marie found that the most noticeable benefit of Reishi was its influence on her insomnia. It not only helped her sleep but also produced a deeper sleep, leaving her more relaxed when she awoke. In Marie's busy schedule she has found that it is her most important supplement. She has stated on many occasions that Reishi is one supplement she feels she will always take.

A Local Retailer's Experience with Reishi

Shelley Peace is the owner/operator of a local health food store called Vega Health Foods. Shelley has a hectic business schedule and at times suffers from shortness of breath and insomnia, especially during peak retail seasons such as Christmas. I introduced Shelley to Reishi as a health supplement, and she began to take it regularly. She soon discovered that her symptoms went away, and now feels better able to handle busy times when she takes Reishi.

This of course stimulated her to mention Reishi to her customers. She recommends it primarily for insomnia and asthma. Many of my patients were also asking Shelley for Reishi and it wasn't long before others on her staff were taking and recommending Reishi. One customer noticed a dramatic improvement in her complexion after using one bottle (Reishi preparations are already used as skin care products in Japan). Vega Health Foods now stocks four types of Reishi products. The mycelium and encapsulated products appear to be the most popular.

Although this pattern may sound like yet another health food fad, most of the Reishi users have noticed significant benefits. Shelley notes that Reishi is now a very important product to her store.

People such as Marie and Shelley have experienced considerable improvement in their lives after consuming Reishi, despite the fact that Reishi's effects are far broader than its reputation as an herb for major illness.

After reflecting on the experiences that others were having with Reishi, I was happy to note that I wasn't the only person using Reishi so intensively in a clinical setting. Once a practitioner added Reishi to their practice, it slowly increased in prominence until it was a major preparation in their repertoire. This was surprising for an herb that was barely used in North America some 2 - 5 years ago.

My own clinical uses, as well as my view of quality control of the product, changed after talking to Michael Broffman and Dr. Dharmananda. It certainly needed to be used in combination, at least with other formulas, or with acupuncture treatments at the same time. Since most practitioners use quite complex programs, with many supplements, this wasn't a problem.

I was also quite pleased to see that others were using Reishi basically as a *Fu Zheng* herb for AIDS and CFS. This is what originally sent me on the search in the first place.

It was obvious to me that its use would increase in the future.

Chapter 8

The Future of Reishi

I had sought out clinical experts in the use of Reishi and a pattern of medicinal uses had become clear. But what of the future of Reishi as a commercial product? What did the designers, manufacturers and commentators in the herbal industry think of this mushroom?

First stop in this task was the West Coast of the United States.

Oregon is a state which has more than its share of supporters. Blessed with great natural beauty and abundant resources, mining, agriculture and logging are all major industries. The combination makes Oregon a place of industrial and natural wealth.

At the south end of the long valley which surrounds the Willamette River lies the well-known university town, Eugene. On the outskirts of town, a small factory produces some of the highest quality herbal extracts in the world. East Earth Herbs is a manufacturer of Oriental and Western herbal formulas used by both alternative health practitioners and the general public.

The owners are Bill and Peggy Brevoort. Peggy was a travelling colleague on my original trip to China with the *People to People* organization. The Brevoorts also have a great place in rural Oregon where I visited them one pleasant summer morning. With their background, it wasn't long before we were discussing Reishi.

Bill has extensive experience in the herb industry, designing and manufacturing formulas that are used around the world.

"Where would you place Reishi in the world of Chinese medicine, Bill?"

"I would consider it very much a `Heart medicine.' This, of course, refers to the physical heart and also the spiritual heart. Reishi is very much a spirit medicine. Some of the myths that surround it say that it takes on the spirit of its surroundings. It is very important that the spirit of the Reishi's surroundings be very `high.'

"This is probably one of the reasons that *Ling zhi* from a deep rain forest area is so valuable, as the deep rain forest contains great spirit. You have to be careful about where the spirit comes from."

"How would you determine the quality of a particular sample of *Ling zhi*?"

"The light *Ling zhi* is not as good as the dark. A good even dark colour is the best, and of course the wild variety is better.

"Over the years we have put great effort into extracting and working with Reishi. Both myself and Qiang Cao, my colleague, have found an alcohol extract to be the best. Water decoctions are good but not as good as the alcohol extraction. This is mainly because the `punch' is in the spores. This oily substance comes out best in alcohol.

"One of the most important ingredients in our *Sage's Ginseng* is a high quality *Ganoderma*. We go to great expense to find the best *Ling zhi* for this product. I won't accept it unless the *Ling zhi* is at least 3/4 spore and, of course, with no insect infestation.

"This formula is meant as a spirit medicine to increase *Sheng Qi* or spiritual essence of the user. We suggest it when the spirit is low from things like too much stress, too much sex, too much friction in life."

"Do you think there are any toxic effects from this herb?" I asked.

"Yes and no. From a Western scientific point of view I would have to say `no.' It is a very safe herb. But the stronger the *Ling zhi*, especially the wild variety, the stronger the reaction on the *Sheng* spiritual body. This of course can bring up a lot of karmic situations for some. People aren't always interested in dealing with old problems."

"Do you mean some kind of spiritual `healing crisis'?"

"Yes, the discharge of karma is going to make people deal with lots of issues. But just like a healing crisis they will awaken to the medicine after a while. This is what I feel some of the so-called side-effects of the mushroom are. We can find this same thing happening with some of the pure wild ginseng. I would have to call these herbs `awareness' medicines, and some people are not interested in awareness."

"Do you think there will be an increase in this herb's popularity in the future?" I inquired.

"Yes I do, but I hope there isn't waste. This is a very special, spirit herb and I hope that it isn't abused. Enough high spirit medicine must be left for the true seeker to use. It is so valuable.

"Some of the great material being released by Subhuti Dharmananda lately will increase its use in San Francisco at least and probably increase its use around the country. It's major value is in increasing *Sheng Qi*.

"In traditional East Indian medicine (Ayurvedic medicine) there are five basic tastes. When listening to a lecture by Dr. Yeshi Donden, the Dalai Lama's physician, he said there was a very special sixth taste that wasn't part of the tradition. It was spirit medicine. It was kind of a bitter, acrid taste. He said that one example is from special mushrooms. *Ling zhi* has this bitter acrid taste, so I would conclude that because of its taste, and some of the history of its use in China, that it would fit into that category."

Bill was yet another person who could tell me something new about Reishi. Was there no end to information on this mushroom? "I am really interested in the subject of *Sheng Qi,*" I said. Some of the myths surrounding Reishi talk about using it to encourage *Sheng Qi.* I've heard of one myth in which mercury was combined to give a special effect."

"Well Terry, I'm not sure that this is just myth. Here in the United States people are taking mercury in combination with secret herbs followed by Reishi, to make the *Sheng Qi* `burn brighter.'"

"But mercury is extremely poisonous!" I exclaimed. "Aren't they worried that they will die? I was told that the First Emperor of China died this very way. With our modern knowledge of mercury I would have thought that everyone would steer clear of it."

"Oh yes! I wouldn't suggest this for the uninitiated," Bill responded.

So the tradition of the Taoists is very much alive, I thought to myself, even here in North America. My visit with the Brevoorts came to an end. I bade my friends goodbye and drove down the road through a beautiful wooded area.

My mind was racing along. You can imagine my excitement. This was at least a partial confirmation that some people have kept alive the old alchemic traditions from the far East. Perhaps some of Dr. Wu's stories were true!

An Editorial View

What about the researchers who watch the North American herb industry? Would they see Reishi's potential? The best person to talk to on this subject would be my good friend Mark Blumenthal.

Mark is the editor and founder of *HerbalGram,* North America's most influential herbal journal. He also writes for many widely distributed consumer health food magazines. This activity makes him a well-known figure in the health food industry, recognized by the professional herbalist and the scientific community.

The board of advisors assembled for *HerbalGram* is most impressive and includes well-known academics, scientists and medical doctors. I first met Mark at a National Health Food Expo, where I was quickly impressed by both his knowledge and his wit. Mark and I have enjoyed many a fine meal over the years and his humorous anecdotes have kept me laughing past the point of comfort on several occasions.

My major interest in talking to Mark was to get the pulse on the trends he saw for Reishi. His position at *HerbalGram* and American Botanical Counsel put him in a key position for timely information. Most information on potential product areas and new developments flows across his desk.

"What kind of experience have you had with Reishi, Mark?" I began.

"Well, to be frank, Terry, I haven't had much personal experience. I have not used it myself or done any personal research on it but I have had lots of second and third hand recommendations. As the editor and publisher of *HerbalGram*, I have seen a lot of research about this herb. Two of the biggest sources were Rob McCaleb's research article on *Ganoderma* that he has produced for *HerbalGram*, and the material produced by Subhuti Dharmananda.

"Apart from the laboratory research, it looks like there is a growing amount of clinical research. We need more of this in the herbal area. The research on Reishi is adding substantially to ideas of how important polysaccharides are in our immune system.

"There is a great deal of research surrounding several plants, such as Echinacea and Astragalus, showing the role of these polysaccharides. I feel this area is quite important."

"Have you seen an increase in information on Reishi in recent years, Mark?"

"Yes. There has been at least a 200-300% increase in this material in recent years, even an increase in recent months."

"Will this trend continue?"

"I would say that the future increase is certain, especially in the AIDS arena with some of the latest clinical research that is coming in from Dharmananda's group. He is using it with AIDS sufferers. I see the whole area of tonics gaining momentum, especially tonics for the immune system. Reishi promises to be a leader in this area. From the information we have been collecting here at *HerbalGram* I can easily say that people are increasing their interest in the quality of their lives, in enhancing their lifestyle. Improvements in the immune system, the first line of defence, increases the realization of this goal."

"Thanks, Mark. I appreciate your overview on Reishi's future."

Mark was a great source for trends in the herbal industry but what about the executives who make decisions for their companies? Had they examined *Ganoderma*?

An International Manufacturer

I decided the next person to talk to was Paul Larsen. His company is one of the largest distributors of herbal products in North America and he has recently added Reishi to his product line. I have worked with Paul for several years, helping with the odd research and development project. I have found his company to have both great integrity and a service ethic. The corporate officers are always watching the current research, looking for important breaking information on botanical products.

"What influenced you to bring Reishi to market, Paul?"

"Well, we keep pretty close watch on what is happening in the scientific community. Steve Bleckman of our parent company, reads all the journals personally. Some of the recent studies are showing promise for both Reishi and Shiitake. We have especially been watching the trend in Japan, where it is being used therapeutically on a significant scale."

"What do you see as the key market niche for medicinal mushroom products?"

"There is no question that the most important niche is immune system enhancement. Current evidence both from lab data and clinical reports is that these mushrooms work on enhancing the immune system. We feel both are important but it looks like Reishi is going to outperform Shiitake as a North American product.

"We are also noticing an increased consumer demand. Even though we are the largest manufacturer in the marketplace with Reishi, we have noticed quite a bit of development in this product area. At the 1989 spring merchandise expo, three marketers carried Reishi. Four months later, at the Summer National show in Las Vegas, 10 marketing companies had a Reishi product on display. I expect increased activity, education and, of course, sales in this area.

"I feel that the polysaccharides in Reishi have stimulated the most interest. Other plants with polysaccharides also have immune enhancing qualities. We believe that Reishi will be used as a single product and in a variety of formulas."

I was getting a pretty consistent picture on how practitioners, manufacturers, and marketing companies were viewing the present and future uses of this mushroom. It seems that Reishi is coming out of the deep dark forest into the limelight of the herb industry. The major interest in Reishi seems to be in its immune system enhancing properties.

A Prominent Researcher

I decided that I should talk to at least one more important figure in the herb industry — Rob McCaleb.

I have also known Rob for several years. He is a key figure in the area of herbal research. Rob McCaleb is the president and founder of the Herb Research Foundation (HRF), which is a "clearinghouse" dedicated to research and education. HRF is a member-funded organization. It presently has approximately 500 members from industry, academia and alternative medicine.

The major task for HRF at this time is bibliographic research. Rob is no newcomer to this industry. He worked in research and development for Celestial Seasonings teas for many years.

Our discussion focused on Reishi, other useful mushrooms and some other polysaccharide-containing products.

Rob began, "There are many fungi that are starting to gain recognition for their medicinal properties. One of special interest that the Japanese call *Polyporus umbellatus* (also known as *Zhu ling* by the Chinese) is showing significant immune modulating abilities. Another, *Enoki* (*Flammulina velutipes* , velvet stem mushroom), is a thin, lanky mushroom which is a very popular edible item. It is interesting to note that within a 150 mile radius of a cultivation area, tumor incidence among humans is significantly lower. Heavy ingestion of *Enoki* is the reputed cause. *O-chawangtake* (*Peziza vesiculosa*) has also shown significant medicinal properties.

"I have seen a significant increase in both the popular press and the scientific literature about medical uses of fungi over the last few years. Information in 1980 was minimal but quite a lot is available now. Probably the most pivotal cause would be research done on the immune system because of AIDS. But we can also see an increase in the amount and variety of edible mushrooms during this same period.

"I see a meaningful increase in the future use of Reishi. At the same time, other mushrooms will increasingly be used as both foods and medicines. Because of the low toxicity and related food uses of mushrooms, I see a favourable regulatory activity in this area. But we do need more research to determine their complete medicinal effects.

"There is a keen interest in this area of research from HRF clients, especially in lentinan extraction from Shiitake.

"The whole area of polysaccharides is of great interest and controversy. Theoretically the polysaccharides should break down before absorption into the human system, converting to simple sugars like glucose. But we know that this can't be happening. For some reason, the polysaccharides are still intact when they reach the bloodstream. Are some of them therefore absorbed by polypinocytosis--a process whereby the cell wall opens for an object? Somehow large molecules can be absorbed into the system.

"Brekhman from the USSR has found that raw sugar also can increase immune function, while white sugar decreases it. Wagner has noted that small doses of Echinacea are often more effective than large doses. Are small amounts of the polysaccharides more significant than large ones? Frankly, Terry, these questions have a lot of people puzzled."

"I have heard some people theorize that reactions on Peyer's Patch in the intestinal tract may be a key factor. If that is true then the substance wouldn't have to be absorbed," I added.

"What role do you see for HRF, for the herbal industry?" I asked.

"I see HRF as a bridge from traditional medicine to modern medicine," he concluded.

I had interviewed a number of scholars from around North America on the clinical and industrial future of Reishi. Will this mushroom become well-known? All this, as Dr. Dharmananda pointed out, has something to do with "fad" promotion. Yet at the same time it was clear that Reishi's healing properties were well-known in the Oriental healing tradition and rapidly gaining recognition among Western medical practitioners.

The stories I had listened to in the Shanghai Sheraton so many months before had been echoed again and again from many different parties.

It was clear that Reishi users, herbal formulators and manufacturers of herbal products shared a common respect for Reishi.

After several thousand years in the confines of Asian pharmacopoeias, Reishi was poised to emerge as a formidable addition to the Western medical armamentarium. It almost seemed as though it had awaited the appearance of such ailments as AIDS, CFS and related immune system deficiencies to signal its entry into battle.

Would it be "Reishi to the rescue!" I chuckled to myself? Maybe the mystical snakes and tigers guarding its location in the deep forest of time had collectively decided that the time was right to reveal the "marvelous herb" to a world deluged by a new wave of life-threatening afflictions. After all, there really are no accidents.

Chapter 9

Dosage and Safety

The Safety of Reishi

I n answer to frequent public concern, Reishi is neither a psychedelic nor toxic. In tests for acute toxicity conducted by Seoul National University in Korea, the water extract of Reishi, after being freeze-dried, showed no lethal or serious side-effects in mice from 5 g/kg (x 70 for people = 350 g) orally for an entire month![66]

Blood, organ weight and body weight showed no changes. Separating a polysaccharide-rich fraction of the water extract, tests in mice with the same dose found essentially the same results.[66]

Reishi syrup was fed to rabbits to find a toxic dose using 4 ml/kg on the first day, 8 ml/kg on the second and 16 ml/kg/day thereafter for the next 7 days, for a total of 140 ml/kg. No toxicity was found. Dogs were administered the syrup at 4 ml/kg and half the dose for the same days. Nothing abnormal could be found except that both kinds of animals ceased to be 'active'. With intragastric administration of a cold-alcohol extract of Reishi in dogs (12 g/kg/day x 15) and a hot-alcohol extract (24g/kg/day x 13), no reactions of a toxic nature were found.[1]

Experiments with rats and numerous toxicity studies with mice also found no signs of toxicity. Young rats intragastrically administered a cold-alcohol extract (12 g/kg/day x 30) showed Reishi had not affected their development, nor did it produce anything abnormal in ECG readings, liver functions or major organs. Similarly, with various mycelial preparations, the level of toxicity from at least 7 studies in China alone was consistently low.[1]

An exception to these animal studies would be allergic reactions. For an indeterminate number of allergic individuals predisposed to mold sensitivities Reishi could conceivably produce an allergic reaction.[49] However, as indicated by the various studies on its anti-allergic properties[37,38,41,42,44,59,60] this remains to be verified using oral doses of Reishi preparations which may in fact produce the opposite reaction, alleviating the symptoms of mold sensitivity.

In clinical studies, side-effects of a severe nature are non-existent and minor ones are few. They include skin rash, loosened stool, dry mouth or a slightly upset stomach, all of which are eliminated by ceasing use of the mushroom and often in the case of digestive problems by taking Reishi with meals.[67]

In our own clinical experience, people with side-effects have them alleviated within a week. (Marie Lefrange noted this in Chapter 7.) These side-effects seem to be a cleansing reaction, often called a 'healing crisis' by Western herbalists.

Finally, large doses, as Dr. Morishige has noted, commonly produce a darkened stool and diarrhea, which he found could be remedied by combining large doses of vitamin C.[52]

Additionally, large doses (10 g/day) of vitamin C are definitely valuable to anyone with cancer[68] or viral diseases.[69,70] However, too much vitamin C can also produce diarrhea. Patients taking vitamin C in doses greater than 10 to 15 grams per day orally (ascorbate powder stirred into a glass of water taken in divided doses, 4 to 6/24 hours) have experienced diarrhea in about 80% of cases.[70]

But if they had a cold, even a mild one, their tolerance to the vitamin increased dramatically with as much as about 50 grams a day producing no diarrhea. In severe colds, twice that and in mononucleosis (caused by the Epstein-Barr virus), influenza or viral pneumonia, 3 times that amount (150 grams/day) is bowel-tolerated.[70]

It seems that the vitamin C the body needs to fight a disease or other condition is taken from the gastrointestinal tract until the required amount is reached. If significantly more than is needed remains, it makes its way to the rectum where it will produce diarrhea.[70]

Dosage and Preparation

Throughout the preceding chapters on Reishi's use in folk-medicine, and the activity studies in China, Japan and Korea, a variety of doses are apparently efficacious, with higher doses being used in the treatment of more life-threatening diseases. Typically, 9 grams a day is used in the treatment of heart diseases or hypertension and in cancer. However, 9 to 15 grams a day in equally divided doses is the rule of thumb.[32]

For Caucasians, who generally weigh more than the Oriental, the higher doses may be advisable. For less serious diseases a smaller amount of Reishi is used. Dosages vary, but approximately 3 to 6 grams a day is generally regarded efficacious in everything from bronchial asthma to insomnia, hepatitis, nervousness and neurasthenia.[32]

More serious diseases, along with mushroom poisoning and pro-longed diseases of the stomach, are treated with higher concentrations of Reishi. One instruction for stomach diseases calls for 90 grams of chopped-up fruit body allowed to soak in half a liter of rice wine for 10 days, after which 60 ml (one fluid ounce) is to be taken two times daily. In mushroom poisoning a 120 gram decoction is prepared, whereas in nervousness and insomnia a 1.5 to 3 gram decoction is made, to be taken twice daily.[32]

A method for preparing decoctions of Reishi and other polypores is found in Kosai Matsumoto's *The Mysterious Reishi Mushroom* (Wood-bridge, 1979). He gives the daily dosage as 2 to 5 grams of dried fruit body per liter of water and suggests that preferably the dried mushroom be reduced to a powder before decocting, the Reishi powder to be placed in a bleached cotton bag. This would eliminate the need for straining but probably wouldn't provide as strong a decoction.

Matsumoto gives the ratio of 2 to 5 grams to a liter of water, and for other polypores 20 grams to 1.8 liters of water. Polypore powders or pieces are decocted at low heat for over 2 hours. One can strain off the decoction and add more water, repeating the process until the water no longer turns color. Reishi is decocted at low heat — just enough to begin bubbling and until the bubbling stops and the volume of water has reduced by two-thirds.[71]

Stronger decoctions are prepared by simply increasing the amount of fruit body to water. For instance, at the ratio of 5 grams per liter of water, the 120 gram decoction used to treat mushroom poisoning would call for 24 liters of water, which is over 6 gallons. For most people, this would require making separate decoctions of a gallon each, 20 grams of fruit body at a time. Using 1/4 the amount of water would provide you with a decoction roughly 4 times the strength in half the time.

How many hours does one keep the decoction simmering? This will be determined by the reduction of water to a third of what you started with. Otherwise, for deliberately longer decoctions, which are bound to be increasingly more potent, simply add more water as needed so as not to scorch the material. Finally, in anticipation of a common inquiry, vitamin C cannot be added during the decoction because heat readily destroys the vitamin.

Conclusion

A Pause in the Journey

Another work day was over. The supper dishes were cleared from the table, replaced by yet another pile of photocopies, files, and my trusty laptop computer. An evening of writing and research lay ahead, but I needed a short break before starting into the material. Through the picture window to the west the sunset was a pink glow over the distant Rockies.

On impulse I went out onto the balcony to catch the warming rays of the sun before the chill of evening set in. The mountains on the horizon were old and beloved companions. It was easy to understand why mountains became sacred to so many cultures. Majestic, basked in clouds and supernatural light, mountains would surely be the realm of gods and immortals.

Writing about Reishi had taken me many miles from home. The foothills of the Rockies were thousands of miles from the crowded streets of Shanghai, hundreds of miles from the Sunshine Coast and the many outstanding professionals who had shared some of their time with me. Yet here I was, in familiar surroundings, needing to bring my experiences together.

Reflecting on the research that had taken me approximately eighteen months to gather, I realized just how far I had come, in distance and in respect for the Reishi mushroom. It had become a major herb in my clinic, as it was in many others throughout North America.

Was Reishi really an "herb of spiritual potency?" Some people certainly believed so. There was no doubt, however, that it was an herb of "medical wonder." Problems relating to the immune system are allopathy's toughest challenge. *Fu Zheng* therapy, of which Reishi is an important part, seems a partial answer to this challenge.

Building up *Wei Qi*, our body's own "military force" — a force more electromagnetic than physical — is a concept with medical utility for us in the West. Several herbs, most of which contain long chain polysaccharides, stimulate this energy. Besides this electromagnetic influence, there is dramatic proof that these herbs have significant biochemical and cellular action. Reishi is certainly a *Fu Zheng* herb, but it so much more.

The ability to inhibit viruses and bacteria, all the while enhancing immune function, insures Reishi a prominent place in any herbalist's repertoire. Add to that its reported effects on cancer and Reishi becomes impossible to ignore. Although these attributes are shared by other polysaccharide-containing plants, mushrooms seem to have a special stature.

The triterpenes and adenosine in Reishi help to explain many this mushroom's effects and potential uses. These compounds impart a cardiovascular cleansing and tonic effect, as well as an adaptogenic boost. A plant such as Reishi could be beneficial for a myriad of our society's most crucial health problems. But it doesn't stop there.

Reishi also alleviates allergies, inhibits Candida, is specific for asthma, squelches free radicals, protects against X-rays, modulates diabetes, regenerates the liver and protects people from elevation sickness. It is no wonder that the ancient Taoists held Reishi in such high esteem, even to the point of reverence.

But I now feel that Reishi's most significant health benefit is its calming action. By putting people into a relaxed state — some have described it as almost meditative — Reishi helps alleviate many of the aforementioned problems. Just the idea of disease can debilitate individuals as much as the disease itself. Almost every health-care practitioner has seen cancer patients wilt at the mere mention of the disease.

It is, therefore, easy to understand why so many myths have sprung up around Reishi. Because this herb works at the basic level underlying many health problems, namely stress, it becomes obvious that its reputation as a longevity plant is well founded. This "mushroom of immortality" reduces the frictions of life that increase aging.

So although I had found many answers to my travels and research, some questions remained. Has Reishi's "spiritual strength" come down from the sacred mountain of the ancient Taoists to aid us at this important historical crossroad, when Western society's health problems seem insurmountable? Will Reishi help direct us towards a new medical theory, one that encompasses both Eastern and Western concepts?

These questions can only be answered by the passage of time. One thing I know for sure. This herb has special healing gifts which we have only begun to investigate. The growing popularity of Reishi in clinics all over the world will bring it to the public eye. The "herb of spiritual potency and medical wonder" is just beginning a new chapter in its long and illustrious history.

Appendices

Reishi Mushrooms in Perspective

They seem to come out of nowhere. In areas where there was no visible sign of their presence, they suddenly appear. Overnight, or so it seems. Such is the nature of mushrooms, the higher order organisms of the world of fungi. Everyone has had some encounter with mushrooms growing in nature. Whether on a walk through the woods, strolling through the park, or just finding them in our lawns and gardens, mushrooms are a phenomenon of nature that cannot be overlooked.

In North America we tend to be somewhat fearful of mushrooms, and generally regard them as something to be avoided. There are, after all, mushrooms that can kill those trusting souls who gather them for the evening's meal. And although we all know someone who is knowledgeable about wild mushroom identification and who regularly picks them with a keenness that borders on the religious, we still keep our distance and play it safe.

This attitude is sharply contrasted by other cultures. Europeans, East and West, are wild about mushrooms and hunt them with a passion. It is said that during the mushroom season in Russia the trains out of Moscow are literally packed with people off to the woods to find their favourite species. In Asia it is no different. Wild and cultivated mushrooms fill the markets and are looked upon with great favor. And nowhere are they so highly prized than Japan. With approximately 12 species cultivated for the marketplace, the Japanese surely lead the world in their appreciation of edible mushrooms. A case in point is the huge volume of pine mushrooms that are now exported from North America to Japan. The highest quality pine mushrooms retail for $500 per pound in Japan and are often bought as gifts or to be savoured on special occasions.

And although their use as food is the most obvious way mushrooms have been used by human cultures, the use of mushrooms as medicine could be the most important contribution these organisms have to make.

Unbeknownst to North Americans except for a handful of researchers and scholars, certain mushrooms have been used as herbal medicines for thousands of years in Japan and China. These mushrooms were some of the most potent, yet benign of the plants that formed the Oriental herbal tradition. Reishi was so highly revered that whole mythologies were built around it, and representations of Reishi can be found throughout Oriental art. So why haven't we heard more about them? For the most part these mushrooms were rare and therefore expensive. In the case of Reishi, only in the past 20 years has it been successfully cultivated. And it is cultivation that has given rise to greater availability for general use and research.

So what actually is a mushroom? Specifically it is a plant that lacks chlorophyll, the substance that green plants use to synthesize food from the sun's energy. A mushroom gets its nutrients from organic matter. And unlike green plants which absorb CO_2 and give off oxygen, mushrooms absorb oxygen and give off CO_2. Mushrooms should be thought of as nature's decomposers — organisms that recycle all the dead animals and plants that accumulate during the course of a normal life and death cycle. Without mushrooms, and other fungi, the Earth would be awash in plant and animal debris. Our soils would not be replenished with fresh humus and our forests would be piled high with leaves, branches, and fallen logs. A world without mushrooms would be a very different place indeed.

As decomposers, mushrooms are separated into three distinct groups. Those that live on dead organic matter, such as leaves, wood wastes, grasses and plants are called saprophytes. Reishi and Shiitake are both saprophytes. Other mushrooms attack living organisms and are termed parasites. A good example would be the honey mushroom, *Armillaria mellea*, a mushroom that kills trees. And the third group are those that form a mycorrhizal relationship with a living plant. These mushrooms form around the roots of plants and trees, providing nutrients to the tree that are otherwise relatively unavailable to it. The mushroom in turn gains nutrients and moisture from the tree rootlets. A mycorrhizal relationship is also termed a symbiosis — a relationship in which two organisms are mutually beneficial partners.

Most mushrooms are composed of a cap and a stem. The underside of the cap has many thin blades radiating out from the central stem. These blades are called gills and are the spore-bearing surface of the mushroom. Spores are the "seeds" by which mushrooms can spread to new areas. The stem lifts the cap above its environment and enables the spores to be carried away by the wind. The Shiitake is an example of this classical mushroom shape.

Not all mushrooms are so classically formed. Polypores, the group to which the Reishi belongs, do not have gills and in many cases lack a stem. The underside of a polypore cap is composed of a tightly packed layer of pores. It is the inside surface of these pores where the spores are propagated. Polypores, commonly known as bracket or shelf fungi, are conspicuous mushrooms that grow off the sides of trees. On a walk through the forest one can commonly see many such bracket mushrooms.

What is not readily visible to us however is the actual mushroom organism, or mycelium. Just as an apple is the fruit of an apple tree, so too is a mushroom the fruit body of a mycelial "tree." Mycelium is a network of fine threadlike filaments that originates from spores. The mycelium spreads throughout the nutrient base or substrate, amassing nutrients as it grows. As long as environmental conditions are right, the mycelium will continue to grow and propagate until it exhausts the available nutrients.

As long as nutrients are available, the mycelium can be considered perennial and will live for many years. At least once a year, mushrooms emerge from the mycelial network. As the reproductive organ of the fungus, mushrooms are the means by which spores are created and spread, thus ensuring the continued existence of the organism.

Mycologists (those trained in mushroom physiology and taxonomy) have devised a system of classification for mushrooms to differentiate the thousands of different species. This classification system enables us to name the various Reishi species that are currently recognised as having medicinal properties. I will also include some of the other mushroom species mentioned in the body of this book.

During a recent trip to China to attend the International Symposium on Mushroom Biotechnology (Nov. 89), I had the good fortune to meet Dr. Ruey-Shyang Hseu, a specialist in Reishi mushroom taxonomy. He was in China specifically to sort out the *Ganoderma* classification system. I had many conversations with Dr. Hseu and was able to accompany him to Beijing to see noted mycologist Dr. Zhao Ji-ding. Dr. Hseu's mission, aside from delivering a lecture on his research at the symposium, was to look at the collection of type specimens collected by Dr. Zhao over his 50 year career. It is only through the preservation of original mushroom material that taxonomists can at a later date check initial classification decisions.

Ganoderma lucidum : The *Ling zhi* or Reishi

The classical Reishi mushroom, *G. lucidum,* has a circular kidney-shaped cap divided by concentric growth rings and resembling a ram's horn. The cap color is a shiny, lacquered red to reddish-brown. It has a creamy white to yellow outer edge when young, which is the newest growth. The distinctive woody stem is attached to one side rather than in the center and is commonly the same color as the cap. The underside is covered with a white pore layer that becomes light brown with age. The sporeprint is brown.

G. lucidum is a wood decomposer that is generally saprophytic although in some cases is parasitic. It grows on deciduous trees and stumps, especially oaks and chestnuts. Its distribution is worldwide, generally fruiting in the warmer areas of the temperate zones in late summer and fall. Another red Reishi that comes up often in the literature is *Ganoderma capense.*

Now that *Ganoderma lucidum* is being cultivated, it should be noted that the mushroom's form is dependent on cultivation conditions. Mushrooms grown on a horizontal surface will have the classic rams horn shape and normal stem. Mushrooms grown on a vertical surface will be more fan shaped with little to no stem. Antler shapes are grown by raising the CO_2 levels in the cultivation room.

Ganoderma tsugae: *Song shan shu zhi*

This mushroom belongs to what polypore specialist at the University of Arizona, Dr. R.L. Gilbertson, calls the "*Ganoderma lucidum* complex" and it is a close look-alike to *G. lucidum*. The cap is reddish-orange with a shellacked appearance. The pore layer is white when young, turning yellow to brown with age. The sporeprint is brown. The stem is attached laterally and has a color similar to the cap. *G. tsugae* grows mainly on conifer trees and only rarely on hardwoods, a distinct difference from *G. lucidum*. It also has a more yellow pore layer and grows at lower temperatures. Its common Chinese name (listed above) means "pine/fir tree fungus."

Ganoderma sinense: *Zi zhi*

Ganoderma sinense has a shiny purplish-black to black cap that grows in concentric rings from the laterally attached black stem. The stem can often grow quite long, as much as 6-8 inches. The cap is kidney-shaped and the new growth at the margin of the cap is pale yellowish brown. The pores are dirty white, turning brown with age. The sporeprint is light brown.

Some mycologists consider this mushroom synonymous with *Ganoderma japonicum*, another black Reishi. However, recent conversations with Dr. Hseu of Taiwan have thrown the existence of *G. japonicum* into doubt. The type species, deposited in Japan, has been lost and without it this species no longer exists scientifically. It may in fact have been *G. sinense*, or what is now being called *Ganoderma neo-japonicum* by Dr. Hseu. *G. neo-japonicum* has a dark purple to black cap and grows on bamboo stumps and roots. Another black species is *Ganoderma formosanum*, which grows on maple trees.

Ganoderma applanatum : The Ancient *Ling zhi*

The Ancient *Ling zhi* is a classical stemless shelf mushroom that grows laterally from dead trees and stumps. It has a brown cap with distinctive semicircular growth rings. The newest growth at the margin of the cap is creamy to light brown in color, turning brown as the mushroom matures. The underside is very white, with a light brown cast in age. The sporeprint is cocoa brown. Known in North America as the "Artist's Conk," the pore layer turns a dark brown when scored, which allows for creative designs to be etched in this surface. *G. applanatum* often survives for more than a single season, with new growth sprouting from the pore layer to form overlapping layers.

A wood decomposer, *G. applanatum* grows on dead deciduous trees and infrequently on conifers such as Hemlock. It is a semi-abundant mushroom distributed worldwide in the Northern temperate zones. This mushroom can grow very large and weigh as much as 5 kg.

The Ancient *Ling zhi* derives its name from the Chinese, *Chih se lao mu chun*, which translates to "flesh colored ancient life source mushroom."

Ganoderma oregonense:

G. oregonense has a reddish brown to dark purple-brown cap with a laterally attached stem of the same color. It has a shellacked, smooth cap and can grow to be very large. Its flesh is thick and less dense than the other *Ganoderma* species. *G. oregonense* grows on conifer trees in Northern California and the Pacific Northwest. Although no work has been done on the medicinal properties of this species, there is every reason to believe that it contains compounds similar to the other Reishi mushrooms.

Lentinus edodes: Shiitake

Young Shiitake mushrooms have a dark reddish brown cap which becomes lighter as the mushroom matures. The cap has fine white threadlike tufts or "scales" on it, especially toward the edges. The gills are white to off white and often have serrated edges. A Shiitake sporeprint is pure white. The stem is typically short and very tough, is centrally attached, and is a dull white to dingy brown color.

The Shiitake is a wood decomposer commonly growing on dead deciduous trees. It derives its name from its association with the *shiia* tree, but also grows well on oak, maple, alder, chestnut and beech. Shiitake is indigenous to Japan, China and other countries in the temperate zone of Indo-China. It typically fruits in the spring and fall.

Polyporus umbellatus: Zhu ling

Zhu ling is a unique mushroom that has multiple light brown to grey caps arising from numerous thin, branched white stems. Often possessing hundreds of small caps and weighing as much as 4 kg, it resembles a dark and fleshy cauliflower. The caps are thin fleshed with a central depression and minute scales that are darker than the general cap color. The underside of the caps are covered with a white pore layer. The sporeprint is white.

Zhu ling is a wood decomposer, arising from a black subterranean sclerotium (a resting stage composed of densely compacted mycelium) at the foot of old deciduous trees and stumps, specifically oaks and beeches. It is widely distributed across the entire northern temperate zone and grows particularly well in warmer areas during the late summer and fall. *Zhu ling* is one of the few polypores that is truly edible and is considered a choice morsel by wild mushroomers. In Chinese herbal medicine it is the sclerotium that is used.

A similar mushroom also noted for its medicinal properties is *Polyporus frondosus*.

Coriolus versicolor: Kawaratake or *Yun zhi*

C. versicolor is a small fan-shaped mushroom that grows laterally in multi-tiered clusters from dead trees. The cap color varies greatly but is generally brown to red-brown, or grey to greenish. It has distinct growth rings that emanate from the center and are of lighter color at the outer margin. The surface of the cap is covered with fine hairs or fibrils which give it a velvety texture. The underside is covered with minute pores that are whitish, becoming light brown to yellowish with age. The sporeprint is whitish. There is little or no stem. The flesh of *C. versicolor* is whitish and leathery. One of the most common polypores, *C. versicolor* is found growing on stumps and fallen trunks and limbs of hardwood trees. Its distribution is worldwide.

Commonly known in Japan as *kawaratake* (mushroom by the river bank) and in China as *Yun zhi* (cloud fungus), *Coriolus versicolor* is one of the first medicinal mushrooms to have an active compound extracted from it and prescribed as a drug. That compound is called PSK (polysaccharide Kurhea). Recently, researchers in Shanghai have produced a new compound from *C. versicolor* called PSP (polysaccharide peptide) which is reputed to be 4 times more potent than PSK and very active against cancer.

Overview

It is now well established that all of the *Ganoderma* species contain polysaccharides and triterpenoids. And yet, the Chinese herbalists assigned different properties to the different Reishi mushrooms. They distinguished the species by color. Recent analytical research would indicate that indeed there are varying quantitative levels of the active components and differences in their occurrence. At the International Symposium on Mushroom Biotechnology (Nanjing, PRC, 1989), I had conversations with Dr. Ching-hua Su of the Taipei Medical College, who reported on his work with triterpenoid analysis of *Ganoderma* species. He stated that all of the *Ganoderma* species he tested contained triterpenoids and that these compounds characterized the genus. He was able to show that each species had a characteristic triterpenoid "fingerprint." Some species contain a broader spectrum of triterpenoids however. And even within a species, different strains will produce varying amounts of specific triterpenoids. Dr. Su indicated that certain triterpenoids were responsible for Reishi's action on specific diseases. He went on to say that a triterpenoid standard was established in Japan due to the ease with which these tests could be run. He is currently working on Reishi polysaccharides and believes they are more important to the action of this mushroom. In fact, the consensus of those I spoke with at the symposium confirmed his thoughts on mushroom polysaccharides.

Mushroom polysaccharides are now the subject of intense research in the Orient. There are upwards of 100 medicinal mushroom products in China, many of which are polysaccharide based, some of which are actual pharmaceuticals. There is a definite shift away from the raw herb and into extracts and mycelial products, both of which can be produced under strictly controlled hygienic conditions. Mycelium production bypasses the time consuming mushroom growing stage. Mycelium, already high in polysaccharides, can be stimulated through the growth media to produce even higher levels. One step away from the pharmaceutical process, the production of mushroom mycelium yields a consistent and clean product.

The Symposium on Mushroom Biotechnology highlighted just how different the Chinese view of mushrooms is from our own. The fact that herbal medical practitioners incorporated mushrooms into the herbal pharmacopoeia is an adventure in itself. That these mushrooms are still highly revered and are continuing to be refined is a testament to a tradition that is gaining strength. China is about to break into the world arena and it may very well be that herbal medicine will be her greatest gift to the world.

contributed by J.S. Chilton

Triterpenes and Sterols

Terpenes take their name from the "turp" in turpentine. Found in oily substances (essential oils), resins and saps of plants, the fragrance of pine and of citrus owes to their terpenes. Pinene (turpentine) and limonene are among the more commonly known.

Triterpenes are found in Siberian ginseng (*Eleutherococcus senticosus*) [47](Please see Notes for Chapter 4) and in Gotu Kola (*Centella asiatica*), two of the more renowned longevity herbs of the Orient. The medicinal activity of Gotu Kola, a creeping herb that grows close to the ground, is mainly found in triterpenes known as "asiaticosides." Applications of the herb in the traditional medicine of China bear obvious similarity to Reishi, being primarily used to treat the respiratory tract and as a blood tonic applied in fevers. Sedative and immuno-enhancing activities offer further similarities.[48]

According to Daniel B. Mowrey, Ph. D., in his highly recommended *Guaranteed Potency Herbs: Next Generation Herbal Medicine* (Cormorant Books, Lehi, Utah, 1988), many are the tales of 100-year-old and older Gotu Kola ingesters in the regions where it grows: Pakistan, Madagascar and India. In Chinese folk-history, a herbalist named Li-Ching Yun is said to have attained a life-span of 256 years from partaking of the herb. Mowrey reports that in Sri Lanka, Gotu Kola and plants with similar activity are regarded as longevity agents — Gotu Kola for the fact that elephants enjoy it and live for so long.[48] The herb is also cooked and eaten raw in salads.[49]

Triterpenes also occur in soybeans in the form of saponins.[50] From the Latin *sapo* meaning soap, saponins foam when shaken. By vigorously shaking an herb tea you can watch for the amount of foam produced to get some idea of the saponin content. Odd as it may seem, soybeans are listed in ancient herbal records for use in treating inflammation and counteracting the aging process.[51]

There are triterpenes in "Hoelen" (*Poria cocos* Wolf)[52], a fungus that grows on pine roots in China where in ancient times adepts in search of longevity or immortality frequently ingested the growth.[53] Also known to Chinese herbalists today as "Fu-ling," *Poria cocos* is the one fungus most frequently used in Oriental herbal formulas where it is found in 30% of prescriptions.[54]

Fu-ling protected mice from the formation of stress-induced ulcers, and taken orally caused a remarkable inhibition of contact dermatitis. But for the most part, Fu-ling remains an enigma to pharmacologists who are at a loss to find a "chemical rationale" to explain its uses in folk-medicine. These include antispasmodic, diuretic and promoting stomach function, and although the fungus has shown only weak antitumor action, anticancer applications as well. [50] On the other hand, the mycelium has significant antitumor activity owing to immuno-modulating polysaccharides. [51,52]

Fu-ling is one of the elixir plants of the ancient Taoists and was classed as a "superior" medicine, meaning it is a substance that brings ease to the body and prolongs life.[138]

This same fungus also grows in North America where it was a survival food for the natives. The early settlers called it "Indian bread," while the Indians called it `tuckah,' `tawking,' `tuckahoe' and similar names. Tuckahoe have the appearance of petrified Irish potatoes, or in their larger forms, of bizarre-looking coconuts. These are tuberous growths with a rough textured extremity and white insides. Technically known as *sclerotia*, they grow under the soil surface where they propagate by living off tree roots and buried or sunken wood. [139] Beneath its stem Reishi also forms a sclerotia which is collected in the wilds of China for use in herbal formulas to treat lung problems.

While *Poria cocos* is a longevity plant in the East, it was of parallel importance in the West where the American Indian used the Fu-ling as a food in times of scarcity. A week's supply of food could be obtained with one day's gathering of tuckahoes, which have a flavour similar to potatoes. Hard as wood when dug up, the Indians softened them by burying them under the heat of a fire. Sliced and sun-dried, their tuckahoes were then ready for grinding and mixing with "sorrel and meal" to make bread. [139]

Similar triterpenes occur in a relative of Fu-ling called Chaga — the renowned "birch tree fungus" (*Poria obliqua* Bres. or *Inonotus obliquus* (Pers. ex Fr.) Pilat)[57,58] which is used as a blood purifier, regenerating agent and cancer cure in the popular medicine of Russia.[59] This fungus was the subject of animal experiments by Michigan State University and the Sloan-Kettering Institute for Cancer Research from 1956 to 1957 when, much as a recipe from Russian folklore prescribed, only an extract made by prolonged decoction — not steeping the fungus as in making tea — would affect tumors.[60]

Clinical application of Chaga preparations in Poland found nearly 20% of patients with third and fourth stage malignancies showed improvements, though predominantly in women with cancer of the genitals or breast. Hard tumors became softer and smaller, pain lessened, hemorrhaging decreased and patients experienced improved sleep and appetite and reported generally feeling better.[61] Investigations in the U.S. and in Finland determined significant antitumor activity in Chaga's triterpenes.[57,58]

The early isolation of triterpenes from The Ancient *Ling zhi* growing in the U.S. was funded in part by a grant from the National Cancer Institute.[62] Despite more recent work with *G.applanatum* [63] and *G. lucidum* triterpenes, to date, none have shown antitumor activity.

An in-depth discussion of this aspect of Chinese herbal medicines is given by Stephen Fulder, Ph. D., in his book *The Tao of Medicine: Oriental Remedies and the Pharmacology of Harmony.* (Destiny Books, 1987.) Fulder presents a "hormone-tuning model" to explain the traditional use of Ginseng as a restorative agent rather than an "instant cure." This amounts to a harmonizing of the actions of the glands which both secrete and are affected by hormones in response to stress from the environment.[68] He explains that triterpenoids are regarded as analogous to the steroids in the body of man and beast (e.g., cholesterol, oestrogen, testosterone, cortisol which controls sugar metabolism and aldosterone which controls water levels in the body), and that chemically they are closely related.[69] But this is not to imply that Ginseng and *Ganoderma* are interchangeable. Contrary to *Ganoderma*, Ginseng can raise the blood pressure. Accordingly, Ginseng is not recommended for those with high blood pressure or a reading of over 180/90.[47]

Fulder senses that "it is more than coincidence that the active principles of most of the harmony remedies are triterpenoids"; that their chemical structure is so reminiscent of steroids should be telling us something more. The effects of hormones on improving sensory awareness, memory, learning and relearning with less errors are improvements of the same kind as those noticed with the triterpenoidal plant-remedies. Fulder found a link through the element of stress, which is consistently less and in some cases far less taxing with these triterpene-containing herbs. Experiments with literally thousands of animals have shown that resistance to all manner of stress is increased and that the ability of these herbs to "restore harmony" is made evident in the presence of greater stress.[70]

The effect of Ginseng on the hormonal response to stress is the main focus of Fulder's hypothesis. If Ginseng increases both the responsiveness of the adrenal glands and their ability to stop excreting when the stress has stopped, their work is conserved, they recover faster and the body is subjected to less adrenaline. Fulder proposes that because of the similarity of the triterpenoids to the body's hormones, they are able to occupy and act in the same sites of action, which is almost everywhere in the body. Because of this the glands would have to manufacture less to achieve the same effect. Put another way, the triterpenoidal herbs "amplify" their effects.

Fulder went on to initiate the first experiments ever conducted to determine whether Ginseng acts on the hypothalamus — the hormone command center where the response of the mind mediates the release of hormones in the body.[140] If his hypothesis was going to prove out there would be no better place to look. The first experiments found that true to his deductions, Ginseng caused the area where the hypothalamus resides — "the lower brain that regulates and monitors internal harmony" — to be immensely sensitized.[70]

Because it is only when stressful situations arise that these kinds of herbs function to aid the body in adjusting to or harmonizing with the environment, Soviet scientists decided to name them "adaptogens." Fulder's "harmony drugs" have essentially the same meaning.[70] The term "adaptogenic" was devised in 1958 by N.V. Lazarev, given to describe the effects of "dibazol," a narcotic that increased the non-specific resistance of an organism to adverse influences." Ten years later Drs. I.I. Brekman and I.V. Dardymov reasoned this sort of action was already common in folk-medicine and later followed their hunch with a survey. Of 189 medicinal plants prescribed in Southeast Asia, those conforming to this action prevailed in herbal formulas used in the treatment of anemia, atherosclerosis, cancer, diabetes, hypertension, "and some other diseases." Particularly noted was their ability to stimulate "production of immune bodies."[71]

Today we have scarcely more than a partial understanding of the activity and mechanisms of adaptogens.[72] Considering that to qualify under this category a substance must be innocuous, causing only a minimum interference with bodily functions, it's no wonder why. And although an adaptogen may have a regulatory or "normalizing" action, as a stiffer requirement it must also enhance resistance to health endangering influences, whether of a chemical, biological or physical nature.[71]

Brekman and Dardymov decided Siberian ginseng and its close relative *Panax ginseng*, conformed to every specification of "adaptogen." These took first and second place in all of the 189 medicinal plants examined. Activity studies showed positive effects in animals from both Ginsengs against effects of radiation, fatigue, and narcotics. For reasons unknown, protection against the toxic effects of anticancer drugs was stronger and more consistent from Siberian ginseng than *Panax ginseng*.[71]

The triterpenes in Ginseng are closely related to a triterpenoid found in the resin of "dammar" or resin trees (*Agathis* species) of New Zealand, New Guinea and the East Indies, and so they are called "dammarane-type" triterpenoids.[69] Those in *Ganoderma* are made up of highly oxygenated lanostane-type triterpenoids.[64,73] Including sterols, oxygenated compounds in *G. lucidum* so far total at least 41 different species.[64] The lanostane types are similar to and therefore take their name from lanosterol, a sterol occurring in the wool-grease of sheep. Lanosterol is also the main precursor or "parent steroid" found in animals,[74] a fact which may prove of greater significance as Fulder's Hormone Hypothesis and the secrets of this mushroom of longevity unfold in the years ahead.

Adenosine

Exactly how adenosine inhibits the aggregation of blood platelets hasn't been entirely worked out, at least not to a satisfactory conclusion everyone will agree upon.[99](Please see Notes for Chapter 4) But what science has learned in trying to understand it is most intriguing indeed, for the findings point to what is very likely Reishi's most subtle, yet fundamental action.

At the outset, adenosine elevates "cyclic AMP levels" in blood platelets.[127] Cyclic AMP (adenosine 3', 5'-cyclic monophosphate), a derivative of adenosine, is found in almost every one of our cells. It mediates a diversity of signals between cells and as such plays a critical role in maintaining the entire cellular — energy functions of the body. Cyclic AMP also acts as an intermediary for the actions of many hormones which increase or decrease levels of cyclic AMP as required.[124]

Appropriately known as the "second messenger" by which hormones are enabled to "transmit" their effects [125], cyclic AMP and the adenosine derivative ATP (adenosine triphosphate) — the energy source for almost every cellular reaction requiring energy and from which cyclic AMP is made.[126] They are part of what Ernest Lawrence Rossi in *The Psychobiology of Mind-Body Healing* (W.W. Norton, 1986) calls the "second messenger system." This cellular system "transduces mind information" through the nervous system to the glands and the various types of cells that constitute the major organs of the body. Within this matrix, called the "cortical-limbic-hypothalamic-autonomic pathway,"[127] are the various hormonal (neuroendocrine) connections behind modulation of the immune system through the mind and emotions, and as well, those of the still less well-known effects of the immune system on the well-being of the mind and body.[128]

Here, we are at once reminded of stress and the Ginseng-hormonal hypothesis of Stephen Fulder. In fact, adenosine was early on a subject primarily of endocrinology and takes its name from the Greek *adenos* meaning gland.

There are results suggesting that by increasing the level of cyclic AMP in platelets, substances which would normally aggregate platelets are inhibited from doing so. This includes *thrombin*, the body's prime aggregator of platelets, and *vasopression*, the platelet aggregating and smooth muscle contracting hormone from the pituitary gland known to raise blood pressure and to contract the muscle tissue of small vessels and capillaries.

Adenosine is therefore a "vasodilator" — an agent or body substance that dilates blood vessels, thereby increasing the flow of blood, particularly through the small vessels or arteries. This action parallels that of one of the body's most important fatty acids, prostaglandin E1, and suggests smooth muscle contraction and platelet aggregation are directly related.[123] Furthermore, cyclic AMP in fatty tissue is lowered by prostaglandins, whereas in platelets cyclic AMP is increased by prostaglandins.[116]

~~Metaphorically~~ the same suggestion is written in a chemical message from the heart. When the flow of blood becomes ~~insufficient the cells~~ that make up the heart muscle release adenosine.[127] Yet there is also a direct relationship to prostaglandin E1 (PGE1), for by raising levels of cyclic AMP, PGE1 indirectly produces anti-inflammatory effects.[129]

Because adenosine directly assists the body in adapting to stress, this nucleotide would appear to account for a significant portion of Reishi's nature as an adaptogen and would likely explain why the content of ATP — the energy source for cellular reactions and the source of cyclic AMP — showed increased levels in the heart muscle (myocardium) of rats administered the Reishi "Heart Relaxant Tablet".[31]

A potent aggregator of blood platelets, adrenaline, produced by the adrenal glands as part of the body's reaction to stress, is normally buffered by the brain through the production of more adenosine to promote the opposite — relaxed and tranquil states.[130] Caffeine antagonizes the mellowing effects of adenosine and may accelerate adrenaline release.[130,131]

Caffeine and adenosine took part in an investigation of Reishi at the Pharmaceutical Institute at Tohuku University in Sendai, Japan in 1987. Yoshimasa Kasabara and Hiroshi Hikino, one of the world's foremost authorities on Oriental medicines, observed definite pain-relieving (analgesic) and mild muscle-relaxant effects from a water extract of Reishi[132]. They isolated adenosine as "an active constituent," indicating that there may be other constituents in the fungus with similar or adenosine-potentiating action.[131]

After injecting (subcutaneous, "s.c.") mice with a hefty dose of caffeine (30 mg/kg), like most of us the mice moved about in their cages with greater frequency. But if the dose of caffeine was combined with a large dose of adenosine (100 mg/kg), the stimulating effect of caffeine was significantly lessened. In another experiment they found that if mice were first administered adenosine (30 mg/kg, s.c.) and then 30 minutes later injected with a lethal dose of caffeine (400 mg/kg, i.p.), time of death was over 200% longer than for mice without adenosine.[131]

After conducting a variety of tests with adenosine on pain and skeletal muscle responses in mice, Kasahara and Hikino concluded that although pure adenosine produced the same effects with greater intensity, in terms of quality the effects of a water extract of Reishi were the same, whether in relaxing muscles, counteracting the lethal toxicity of caffeine or in reducing pain.[131] The water extract, prepared by boiling the crushed fruit body in water (2 hours) and then freeze drying the remaining liquid, produced a variety of results indicating a definite calming effect on the central nervous system.[132]

Mice injected with caffeine (20 mg/kg, s.c.) and put in wheel cages normally increase the number of revolutions the wheels turn. But when Reishi was administered (300 mg/kg) at the same time as the caffeine, revolutions made were significantly less. Compared to mice given neither caffeine or Reishi, mice administered the mushroom alone (30 mg/kg, s.c.) also made significantly fewer revolutions.[132]

In high single doses, which are used to get an indication of the effects of prolonged use, the Reishi extract (300 mg/kg, s.c.) prolonged the life of mice given a lethal dose of strychnine. In all, ten different tests were performed with the mushroom extract before their conclusion: the reduced spontaneous motor activity in mice was due to a central nervous system calming effect and a relaxant action on muscles.[132]

Adenosine definitely has a role in the medicinal effects of Reishi and will probably also appear in other medicinal herbs once they are examined more carefully.

Table of Active Constituents

Active compound	Compound Type	Action	Species	Plant form	Citation
Cyclooctasulphur		Histamine release inhibitor	G. lucidum	Mycelium	1
**	Alkaloids	Cardiotonic	G. lucidum	Fruit body	2
**	Glycoproteins	Tumor inhibitors	G. species	Fruit body	3
RNA	Nucleic acid	Interferon inducing;anti-viral	G. applanatum	Fruit body	4
Uridine, Uracil	Nucleosides	Neuro-muscular restoratives	G. capense	Mycelium	5
Adenosine	Nucleotide	Blood platelet aggregation inhibitor;muscle relaxant;analgesic			5,7
Ganoderans A,B	Polysaccharide	Hypoglycemic	G. lucidum	Fruit body	9
Ganoderan C	Polysaccharide	Hypoglycemic	G. lucidum	Fruit body	10
**	Polysaccharide	Cardiotonic	G. lucidum	Fruit body	11
G-A(Beta-glucan)	Polysaccharide	Anti-inflammatory	G. japonicum	Fruit body	12
**	Polysaccharide	Anti-tumor; Immunostimulating	G. lucidum	Fruit body	13
Beta-D-glucan	Polysaccharide	Anti-tumor; Immunostimulating	G. lucidum	Fruit body	14
GL-I	Polysaccharide	Anti-tumor; Immunostimulating	G. lucidum	Mycelium	15
Beta-D-glucan G-Z	Polysaccharide	Anti-tumor; Immunostimulating	G. lucidum	Fruit body	16
Beta-D-Glucan	Polysaccharide	Anti-tumor; Immunostimulating	G. applanatum	Fruit body	16
G-I-2a	Polysaccharide	Anti-tumor; Immunostimulating	G. applanatum	Fruit body	17
Beta-D-glucan	Polysaccharide	Anti-tumor; Immunostimulating	G. applanatum	Fruit body	18

** not identified.

Active Constituents (continued)

Active compound	Compound Type	Action	Species	Plant form	Citation
Beta-D-glucans	Polysaccharide	Anti-tumor; Immunostimulating	G. lucidum	Mycelium	14
FA,FI,FI-1a Beta-D-glucans	Polysaccharide	Anti-tumor; Immunostimulating	G. lucidum	Fruit body	19
**	Polysaccharide	Anti-carcinogenic	G. tsugae	Mycelium	20
**	Polysaccharide	Anti-carcinogenic	G. boninense	Mycelium	20
D-6	Polysaccharide	Protein synthesis enhancer; nucleic acid metabolism enhancer			
Ling Zhi - 8	Protein	Broad spectrum anti-allergic; Immunomodulator	G. lucidum	Fruit body	21
Ganodosterone	Steriod	Anti-hepatotoxic	G. lucidum	Mycelium	22
Ganoderic Acids A,B,C-2,D	Triterpene	Histamine Release Inhibitor	G. lucidum	Mycelium	23
Ganoderic Acids R,S	Triterpene	Anti-hepatotoxic	G. lucidum	Fruit body	24
Ganoderic Acids B,D,F,H,K,S,Y	Triterpene	Anti-hypertensive, ACE inhibiting	G. lucidum	Mycelium	25
Ganodermadiol	Triterpene	Anti-hypertensive, ACE inhibiting	G. lucidum	Fruit body	26
Ganoderic Acid Mf	Triterpene	Cholesterol synthesis inhibitor	G. lucidum	Fruit body	26
Ganodermic Acid T-0	Triterpene	Cholesterol synthesis inhibitor	G. lucidum	Mycelium	27
Ganoderic Acid B	Triterpene	Cholesterol synthesis inhibitor	G. lucidum	Mycelium	27
Oleic Acid	Unsaturated fatty acid	Histamine	G. lucidum	Fruit body	28

Glossary

Adaptogen: An adaptogen helps a person increase resistance to a large range of biological, environmental, psychological and chemical stresses. This word and *phannominum* were originally created by Dr. Brekhman in Russia to explain Siberian ginseng's (*Eleuthrococcus senticosus*) action. This word has since been used to explain the functioning of many Fu Zheng type herbs.

Anti-oxidant: Substances that inhibit the action of free radicals that are caused by oxidants. Common examples of anti-oxidants are Vitamins A, C, E, Beta Carotene, Super Oxide Dismutase.

Antigen: Substances that cause allergies.

Candida: A common type of yeast infection.

Chronic Fatigue Syndrome (a.k.a. Chronic Epstein Barr Virus): A disease that might be caused by Epstein Barr virus or many other viruses. Its symptoms include severe fatigue, sore throat, poor concentration, anxiety/depression, headaches, hypersensitivities and allergies.

Fu Zheng: A Chinese therapy that is similar to immune therapy in Western medicine. These therapies include botanical and acu-puncture treatment to increase resistance to disease. (See also *Wei Qi.*)

HDL: High Density Lipoproteins are types of cholesterol that are generally considered good.

Hyperlipidemia: A state representing high levels of fatty acids in the blood.

Hypoglycemic: A state of low levels of blood sugar.

145

Immunoglobulins (IgA,E,G,M): A group of protein molecules important to the body's immunologic system. The letter represents the molecular size. IgG often are activated in digestive allergies, while IgA is often activated in respiratory allergies.

Interferon: A protein that protects a cell membrane from virus attachment.

Karma: An Eastern religious concept stemming from the idea of rebirth. A person pays for wrongdoing in one lifetime in a future lifetime.

LDL: Low Density Lipoprotein is a type of cholesterol which is generally considered bad, as it is the type which is most likely to plaque on arterial walls.

Leukocytes: White blood corpuscles that act as scavengers to help combat infection.

Macrophages: Large cells that have the ability to phagocytose or engulf foreign substances or organisms to aid the body's immune system in fighting infection.

Mycelium: A network of thread-like strands constituting the vegetative body of mushrooms and other fungi.

Phagocytosis: The ability to engulf foreign substances or organism to aid the immune system in fighting infection.

Philosopher's stone: These are stones created through secret methods and rites to create very powerful medicine. There are two basic types: the *little works* or plant stone and the *mineral works* of changing base minerals into philosopher's gold.

Platelet aggregation: The process of platelets gathering into clumps that could cause blood clots, the precursors to strokes, some types of migraines, and thrombi.

Polysaccharides: Very long chains of glucose sugar. Many of the immuno-active polysaccharides are branched in nature.

Qi (Chee, chi): A non physical energy that is theorised in Chinese medicine to flows through acupuncture meridians. Qi is possessed by herbs that in turn impart qi to the human system. The basic substance of the universe. See also *Sheng Qi* and *Wei Qi*.

Sheng Qi: The energy that is possessed by the spirit.

Spawn: The aggregation of mycelium on a carrier material which is usually used to inoculate prepared substrates.

Spore: The reproductive cells or "seed" of fungi.

T-cells: A specific lymphocyte that has matured in the thymus gland.

Taoists: A Chinese religious sect that is based on the concept of Yin (-) and Yang (+) dualistic universe.

Thrombi: A blood clot obstructing a blood vessel.

Wei Qi: A Chinese concept for special type of energy that represents the military or protective forces of the body. Similar to an immune function.

Yang (deficiency): Male, positive, heavenly energy being low in a person.

Yin (deficiency): Female, negative, earthly energy being low in a person.

Notes

Further Reading for Chapter 1

Bretsschneider E.,*Botanicum Sinicum: Notes on Chinese botany from Native and Western Sources. Part I,* Journal of the North-China Branch of Royal Asiatic Society; 1881; New series; 16:(Part One); 224-227.

Bretsschneider E.,*Botanicum Sinicum: Notes on Chinese botany from Native and Western Sources.* Journal of China Branch of Royal Asiatic Society; 1890-1891; New series; 25: 40-41 and 194.

Bretsschneider E.,*Botanicum Sinicum: Notes on Chinese botany from Native and Western Sources. Part III,* Journal of China Branch of Royal Asiatic Society; 1894-1895; New series; 29: 418-420.

Chikashige, M.; *Oriental Alchemy.* Samuel Weiser, New York, 1974; iv-v.

Dubs, H; "The Beginning of Alchemy," *Isis* (1949); 2: 62-86.

Dubs, H; *The History of Former Han Dynasty by Pan Ku;* Volume Two. Waverly Press, Baltimore, 144: 91 and 239.

Davis T.L.; *The Chinese beginning of Alchemy* Endeavour 1943; 2(8): 154-60.

Davis T.L. & Kuo-Fu C., *The Inner Chapter of the Pao-P'u-Tzu"* Proceeding of the American Academy of Arts and Sciences 1938-42; 74 Sect 89-101; 297-327.

Davis T.L. & Lu-Ch'iang Wu, "Chinese Alchemy," *The Scientific Monthly* (1930); 31: 225-235.

Feifel E (translator) *Pao-P'u Tzu Nei-P'ien,* Chapters XI, Monumenta Serica 1946 11:1-32.

Lin Zhi-bi; *The Present Status of Pharmacological Studies of Ling zhi (Ganoderma lucidum in China;* Yao Hseuh Pao 14(3):183-192 1979.

Mahdihassan S; *Indian Alchemy or Rasayana in the Light of Asceticism Geriatrics.* Vikas Pub House, PVT Ltd. New Delhi, 1979; 106, 64-65, 46.

Needham, J. ; *Science and Civilization in China.* Vol. 5 , Part II. Cambridge at the University Press, 1974; 114-123.

Shizhen Ji, *Ben Cao Gang Mu ,* Shang Wu Printer, 1933.

Sivin, Nathan. *Chinese Alchemy: Preliminary Studies.* Harvard University Press, 1968; 108, 181 and 200.

Notes for Chapter 3

Reishi in Cancer Research

1. Toshio Miyazaki and Motohiro Nishijima, "Studies on Fungal Polysaccharides. XXVII. Structural Examination of a Water-Soluble, Antitumor Polysaccharide of Ganoderma lucidum", Chemical and Pharmaceutical Bulletin (1981); 29(12): 3611-3616.

2. Wen-yen-Li and Eric J. Lien, "Fu zhen Herbs in the Treatment of Cancer", Oriental Healing Arts International Bulletin (1986); 11(1): 1-8.

3. Kosai Matusmotto II. The Mysterious Reishi Mushroom. Woodbridge Press Publishing Company, Santa Barbara, California, 1979; 31-42.

4. Ref. 3; 21-22.

5. Ref. 3; 18.

6. Ref. 3; 25.

7. Liu Bo and Bau Yun-Sun. Fungi Pharmacopoeia. The Kinoko Company, Oakland, California, 1980; 199.

8. Tetsuro Ikekawa, Miyako Nakanishi, Nobuaki Uehara, Goro Chihara, and Fumiko Fukuoka, "Antitumor Action of Some Basidiomycetes, especially Phellinus Linteus", The Japanese Journal of Cancer Research (1968); 59: 155-157.

9. S. Tsukagoshi, Y. Hashimoto, G. Fuji et al., "Krestin (PSK)", Cancer Treatment Reviews (1984); 11(2): 131-135.

10. Hitoshi Ito, Sensuke Naruse, and Keishiro Shimura, "Studies on Antitumor Activity of Basidiomycetes Polysaccharides. VII. Antitumor Effect of the Polysaccharide Preparations from Ganoderma lucidum on Mouse Sarcoma 180", Mie Medical Journal (1977); 26(2-3): 147-152.

11. B.K. Kim, H.S. Chung, K.S. Chung and M.S. Yang, "Anti-neoplastic Components of Korean Basidiomycetes", Korean Journal of Mycology (1980); 8(2), from BIOSIS Previews.

12. Byong Kak Kim, Hee Soo Chung, Kyung Soo Chung, Moon Sik Yang, "Studies on the Antineoplastic Components of Korean Basidiomycetes", Hanguk Kyunhakhoe Chi (1980); 8(2): 107-113.

13. Chang Yul Kan, Mi Ja Sim, Eung Chil Choi et al., "Studies on Antineoplastic Components of Korean Basidiomycetes". Mycelial Culture and an Antineoplastic Component of Ganoderma lucidum", Hanguk Saenghwa Hakhoe Chi (1981); 14(2): 101-112, (in Korean), in Chem. Abstr. 95: 144002m.

14. Toshi Miyazaki and Motohiro Nishijima, "Structural examination of an alkali-extracted, water-soluble heteroglycan of the fungus Ganoderma lucidum", Carbohydrate Research (1982); 109: 290-294.

15. Toshio Miyazaki, "Relationship Between the Chemical Structure and Antitumor Activity of Basidiomycetes Glucans", Shinkin to Shinkinsho (1983); 24(2): 95-101, (in Japanese), in Chem. Abstr. 100: 79551v.

16. Takashi Mizuno et al., "Fractionation, Chemical Modification and Antitumor Activity of Water-insoluble Polysaccharides of the Fruiting Body of Ganoderma lucidum", Nippon Nogei Kagaku Kaishi (1985); 59(11): 1143-1151, (in Japanese), in Chem. Abstr. 104: 135927u.

17. Takashi Mizuno, Naomi Kato, Atsushi Totsuka et al., "Fractionation, Structural Features and Antitumor Activity of Water-soluble Polysaccharide from "Reishi", the Fruit Body of Ganoderma lucidum", Nippon Nogei Kagaku Kaishi (1984); 58(9): 871-880, (in Japanese), in Chem. Abstr. 101: 226886j.

18. Yoshiaki Sone, Reiko Okuda, Noriko Wada et al., "Structures and Antitumor Activities of the Polysaccharides Isolated from Fruiting Body and the Growing Culture of Mycelium ofGanoderma lucidum", Agricultural and Biolgical Chemistry (1985); 49(9): 2641-2653.

19. Hea Won Shin, He Won Kim, Eung Chil Choi et al., Studies on Constituents of Higher Fungi of Korea. Part XLIII. Studies on Inorganic Composition and Immunopotentiating Activity of Ganoderma lucidum in Korea", Saengyak Hakhoechi (1986); 16(4): 181-190, (in Korean), in Chem. Abstr. 105: 29874k.

20. Teikoku Chemical Industry Co., Ltd., Mushroom Glycoproteins as Neoplasm Inhibitors, Japanese Patent No. 82 75,926, May 12, 1982, in Chem Abstr. 97: 44311j.

21. Kureha Chemical Industry Co., Ltd., Anticarcinogen, Japanese Patent No. 76 17,166, May 31, 1976, in Chem. Abstr. 85: 170730v.

22. Shoji Shibata, Yoshihiro Nishikawa, Cheng Fu Mei et al., "Antitumor Studies on Some Extracts of Basidiomycetes", The Japanese Journal of Cancer Research (1968); 59(2): 159-161.

23. Liu Bo and Bau Yun Sun, Fungi Pharm, The Kinoko Co. Oakland, CA, 1980, 168-169.

24. Jonathan L. Hartwell, "Plants Used Against Cancer", The Journal of Natural Products (1971); 34(4): 419.

25. Takashi Mizuno, Taichi Usui, Masashi Tomoda et al., "Studies on the Host-Mediated Antitumor Polysaccharides. II. Screening Test on Antitumor Activity of Various Kinds of Polysaccharides", Shizuoka Daigaku Nogakubo Kenkyu Hokuku (1980); (30): 41-50, (in Japanese), in Chem. Abstr. 94: 202749c.

26. Taichi Usui, Yoshio Iwasaki, Katsuyuki Hayashi et al., "Antitumor Activity of Water-soluble Beta-D-Glucan Elaborated by Ganoderma applanatum", Agricultural and Biological Chemistry (1981); 45(1): 323-326.

27. Takashi Mizuno, Masashi Ushiyama, Taichi Usui et al., "Studies on the Host-Mediated Antitumor Polysaccharides. VI. Isolation and Characterization of Antitumor Active Beta-D-Glucan from Mycelial Cells of Ganoderma applanatum", Shizuoka Daigaku Nogakubu Kenkyu Hokoku (1982); (32): 41-58, (in Japanese), in Chem. Abstr. 98: 212585t.

28. Taichi Usui, Yoshio Iwasaki, Takshi Mizuno et al., "Isolation and Characterization of Antitumor Active Beta-D-Glucans from the Fruit Bodies of Ganoderma applanatum", Carbohydrate Research (1983); 115: 273-280.

29. Subhuti Dharmananda, Ph. D. Chinese Herbal Therapies for Immune Disorders. Institute for Traditional Medicine and Preventive Health Care, Portland, Oregon, 1988; 9-35.

30. Martyna Kandefer-Szerszen, Zbigniew Kawecki, and Maria Guz, "Fungal Nucleic Acids as Interferon Inducers", Acta Microbiologica Polonica (1979); 28(4): 277-291.

31. Jong Hyup Kim and Jeong Sook Nam, "Studies on distribution of the mononucleotides in Ganoderma lucidum", Han'guk Kyunhakhoechi (1984); 12(3): 111-116, (in Korean), in Chem. Abstr. 101: 226480x.

32. Hong-Yen Hsu et al, editors. Oriental Materia Medica: A Concise Guide. Oriental Healing Arts Institute, Long Beach, California, 1986; 640-641.

33. Cheng-Chuang Tseng, Hsue-Fen Chen and Hsien-I Tseng, "Preliminary Report of the Hot-Water Extract of Basidiomycetes As Immunogen Against Experimental Escherichia coli Infection in Mice", Journal of the Taiwan Pharmaceutical Association (1981); 33(1): 16-21.

34. Hong Chang Guan and Zheng Cong, "Effects of Ling Zhi polysaccharide D6 on the biosynthesis of nucleic acid protein and its preliminary analysis", Yaoxue Tongbao (1982); 17(3): 177-178, (in Chinese), in Chem. Abstr. 97: 155971u.

35. Shoichi Nakashima, Yukio Umeda, and Taira Kanada, "Effect of Polysaccharides from Ganoderma applanatum on Immune Responses. I. Enhancing Effect on the Induction of Delayed Hypersensitivity in Mice", Microbiology and Immunology (1979); 23(6): 501-513.

36. M.S. Lee and K-S. Chung, "The Effects of Ganoderma lucidum Extracts and Filtrate of Escherichia coli Culture on Leucocyte Chemotaxis", Korean Journal of Mycology (1987); 15(1): 1-8, (in Korean).

37. Donna Y. Muirhead and Gustavo Cudkowicz, "Subpopulations of Splenic T cells Regulating an Anti-Hapten Antibody Response. I. Helper and Amplifier Cells", The Journal of Immunology (1978); 120(2): 579-585.

38. Ian R. Tizard, *Immunology: An Introduction,* Saunders College Publishing, Phila. PA. 1984, pp. 94,323.

39. Fukumi Morishige, Takahide Nakamura, Nakao Nakamura, and Noritsuga Morishige, "The Role of Vitamin C in Tumor Therapy (Human)". In Vitamins and Cancer: Human Cancer Prevention by Vitamins and Micronutrients. Frank L. Meyskens, Jr. and Kedar N. Prasad, editors. Humana Press, Clifton, New Jersey, 1986; 399-427.

40. Becoming Healthy with Reishi, III. Kampo I-yaku Shimbun, Toyo-Igaku Sha Co. Ltd., Tokyo, 1988; 12-20.

Notes for Chapter 4 (and Portions of the Appendices)

1. The Third Hospital of Hong Qiao District in Tianjin. Clinical Observation on Hyperlipemia Treated with Lingzi (Ganoderma) Tablets. Chinese Traditional and Herbal Drugs (1977); (1): 35-36. Fu Kezhi, trans.

2. Robert S. Harris and Kenneth V. Thimann, editors. Vitamins and Hormones: Advances in Research and Applications, VII. Academic Press Inc., New York, 1949; 39.

3. Ronald J. Landry, "Hypertension: Of Thickened Blood and Failing Hearts", American Health (1984); 15.

4. R.C. Robbins, "Effects of Phenyl Benzo-Gamma-Pyrone Derivatives (Flavonoids) on Blood Cell Aggregation: Basis for a Concept of Mode of Action", Clinical Chemistry (1971); 17(5): 433-437.

5. R.C. Robbins, "Effects of Flavonoids on Survival Time of Rats fed Thrombogenic or Atherogenic Regimens", Journal of Atherosclerosis Research (1967); 7: 3-10.

6. Nanjing Branch of ther National Medical Society, Association of Heart Vessels Disease and No. 6 Department of Hunan Institute of Pharmaceutical Industry. Clinical Observation on the Treatment of 103 Cases of Coronary Heart Disease with Ganoderma Shu Xin Tablets, Chinese Traditional and Herbal Drugs (1979); (6): 32-33. Fu Kezhi, trans.

7. Subhuti Dharmananda, Chen Fu Tai, and George Weissmann, "Herbal Foods in Asia: Role in the Prevention and Treatment of Cardiovascular Diseases". In Nutrition and Heart Disease II. Ronald R. Watson, Ph. D., editor. CRC Press, Inc., Boca Raton, Florida, 1986; 96-97.

8. "Lingzhi". Pharmacology and Applications of Chinese Materia Medica, I. Hson-Mou Chang, Ph. D. and Paul Pui-Hay But, Ph. D., editors. World Scientific Publishing Co. Pte Ltd., Singapore, 1986; 642-653.

9. Tsutomu Tamura, Toshio Takahashi and Satoshi Matsuda, "Fermentation product as food additives for patients with hyperlipidemia", (1987); in Chem. Abstr; CA108(13): 110854n.

10. Liu Bo and Bau Yun-Sun. Fungi Pharmacopoeia (Sinica). The Kinoko Company, Oakland, California, 1980; 172.

11. Katsuo Kanmatsuse, Nagao Kajiwara, Kyoko Hayashi et al., "Studies on Ganoderma lucidum. I. Efficacy against Hypertension and Side Effects", Yakugako Zasshi (1985); 105(10): 942-947 (in Japanese).

12. Yearul Kabir, Shuichi Kimura, and Tsutomu Tamura, "Dietary Effect of Ganoderma lucidum Mushroom on Blood Pressure and Lipid Levels in Spontaneously Hypertensive Rats (SHR)", Journal of Nutritional Sciences and Vitaminology (1988); 34(4): 433-438.

13. Michinori Kubo, Hideaki Matsuda, Tadato Tani et al., "Effects of Soyasaponin on Experimental Dissemenated Intravascular Coagulation. I.", Chemical and Pharmaceutical Bulletin (1984); 32(4): 1467-1471.

14. Masaako Ito et al., "Anti-allergic Effects of Reishi (Ganoderma lucidum)". Poster 24. International Congress on Natural Products Research. American Society of Pharmacognosy and Japanese Society of Pharmacognosy. Twenty-ninth Annual Meeting of the American Society of Pharmacognosy, Park City, Utah, July 17-21, 1988. University ___. ___. Of Medicinal Chemistry. Salt Lake City, Utah, 1988.

15. Tsuyoshi Nishitoba, Hiroji Sato, Sachiko Shirasu and Sadao Sakamura, "Novel Interpenoids from the Mycelial Mat at the Previous Stage of Fruiting of Ganoderma lucidum, Agricultural and Biological Chemistry (1987); 51(2): 619-622.

16. Norman R. Farnsworth, A. Douglas Kinghorn, Djaja D. Soejarto and Donald P. Waller, "Siberian Ginseng (Eleuthorococcus senticosus): Current Status as an Adaptogen". In Economic and Medical Plant Research, I.H. Wagner, Hiroshi Hikino and Norman R. Farnsworth, editors. Academic Press, 1985; 155-215.

17. Daniel B. Mowrey, Ph. D. Guaranteed Potency Herbs: Next Generation Herbal Medicine. (1988). Cormorant Books, P.O. Box 386, Lehi, Utah 84043.

18. J.C. Th. Uphof. Dictionary of Economic Plants. Verlag Von J. Cramer, New York, 1968; 118.

19. Isao Kitagawa, Masayuki Yoshikawa, Hui Kang Wang et al., "Revised Structures of Soyasapogenols A, B, and E, Oleanene-Sapogenols from Soybean. Structures of Soyasaponins I, II, and III", Chemical and Pharmaceutical Bulletin (1982); 30(6): 2294-2297.

20. Michinori Kubo, Hideaki Matsuda, Tadato Tani, "Effects of Soyasaponin on Experimental Disseminated Intravascular Coagulation. I", Chemical and Pharmaceutical Bulletin (1984); 32(4): 1467-1471.

21. Jocelyne Valisolalao, Luu Bang, Jean Paul Beck and Guy Ourisson, "Etude chimique et biochimique de drogues chinoises. V. Cytotoxicit@ de triterp@nes de Poria cocos (Polyporacae) et de substances analogues", Bulletin de la Societe Chimique de France (1980); (Part II); 9-10: 473-477.*

*Antitumor polysaccharides only show up in the mycelia of P. cocos.54-56

22. Joseph Needham. Science and Civilization in China, 5(Part 5). Cambridge University Press, 1983; 33.

23. Hiroshi Hikino, "Recent Research on Oriental Medicinal Plants". In Economic and Medicinal Plant Research, I. H. Wagner, Hiroshi Hikino and Norman R. Farnsworth editors. Academic Press, 1985; 53-85.

24. Lemont B. Kier, "Triterpenes of Poria obliqua", Journal of the Pharmaceutical Society (1961); 50(6): 471-474.

25. Kirsti Kahlos, L. Kangas and R. Hiltunen, "Antitumor activity of Triterpenes in Inonotus obliquus", Planta Medica (1986); (6): 554.

26. Alma R. Hutchens. Indian Herbology of North America. Merco, Windsor, Ontario, Canada, 1974; 77-80.

27. E.H. Lucas, "The Role of Folklore in Discovery and Rediscovery of Plant Drugs", Centenial Review (1959); 3: 173-188.

28. Stanislaw Piaskowski, "Preliminary Studies on the Preparation and Application of Preparations from Black Birch Touchwood in Human Cases of Malignant Tumors", Sylwan (1957); 101(10): 5-11 (In Polish).

29. George R. Pettit and John C. Knight, "Steroids and Related Natural Products. XII. Fomes applanatus", Journal of Organic Chemistry (1962); 27: 2696-2698.

30. Jiri Protiva, Hana Skorkovska, Jiri Urban and Alois Vystrcil, "Triterpenes and Steroids from Ganoderma applanatum", Collection of Czechoslovakian Chemical Communications (1980); 45(10): 2710-2713.

31. Sheau-Farn Yeh, Kung-Chi Lee and Ming-Shi Shia, "Sterols, Triterpenes and Fatty Acid Patterns in Ganoderma lucidum", Proceedings of the National Science Council, Republic of China (Part A): Physical Science and Engineering (1987); 11(2): 129-134.

32. Helmut Ripperger and Herbert Budzikiewicz, "Steroid aus Ganoderma applanatum", Phytochemistry (1975); 14: 2297-2298.

33. D. Kac, G. Barbieri, M.R. Falco et al., "The Major Sterols from Three Species of Polyporaceae", Phytochemistry (1984); 23(11): 2686-2687.

34. Stephen Fulder, Ph. D. The Tao of Medicine. Destiny Books, Inner Traditions Int'l., Rochester, Vermont, 1987; 212.

35. Ref. 34; 145-146.

36. Ref. 34; 161-162, 169-171 and 174.

37. I.I. Brekman and I.V. Dardymov, "New Substances of Plant Origin which Increase Non-specific Resistance", Annual Review of Pharmacology (1969); 9: 419-430.

38. H. Wagner and A. Proksch, "Immunostimulatory Drugs of Fungi and Higher Plants". In Economic and Medicinal Plant Research, 1. H. Wagner, Hiroshi Hikino and Norman R. Farnsworth, editors. Academic Press, 1985; 113-153.

39. Lee-Juian Lin, Ming-Shi Shiao, and Sheau-Farm Yeh, "Seven New Triterpenes from Ganoderma lucidum", Journal of Natural Products (1988); 51(5): 918-924.

40. "lanosterol". Dorland's Illustrated Medical Dictionary. Twenty-sixth edition. W.B. Saunders, 1981; 712.

41. Tsuyoshi Nishitoba, Hiroji Sato and Sadao Sakamura, "Novel Mycelial Components, Ganoderic Acid Mg, Mh, Mi, Mj and Mk, from the Fungus Ganoderma lucidum", Agricultural and Biological Chemistry (1987); 51(4): 1149-1153.

42. Masao Hirotani, Isao Asaka, Chieko Ino et al., "Ganoderic Acid Derivatives and Ergosta -4, 7, 22-Triene-3, 6-Dione from Ganoderma lucidum", Phytochemistry (1987); 26(10): 2797-2803.

43. William R. Nes, Ph. D. and Margaret Lee McKean, Ph. D. Biochemistry of Steroids and Other Isopentenoids. University Park Press, 1977; 536.

44. "Sterols". The Harper Encyclopedia of Science. James R. Newman, editor. Harper and Row, 1967; 1137.

45. Masami Miura, Setsuko Onta, Sasahi Kamogawa et al., "Basic Study of Assay Method of Choleretic Effect and the Screening of Crude Drugs", Yakugaku Zasshi (1987); 107(12): 992-1000 (in Japanese).

46. Jonathan L. Hartwell and Betty J. Abbott, "Antineoplastic Principles in Plants", Advances in Pharmacology and Chemotherapy. (1969); 7: 117-209.

47. Robert F. Raicht, Bertram I. Cohen, Eugene P. Fazzini et al., "Protective Effect of Plant Sterols Against Chemically Induced Colon Tumors in Rats", Cancer Research (1980); 40: 403-405.

48. Aiko Morigawa, Katsuaki Kitabatake, Yoshinori Fujimoto and Nobuo Ikekawa, "Angiotensin Converting Enzyme-Inhibitory Triterpenes from Ganoderma lucidum", Chemical and Pharmaceutical Bulletin (1986); 34(7): 3025-3028.

49. Ming-Shi Shiao, Lee-Juian Lin, Sheau-Farn Yeh, and Cheng-Shiang Chou, "Two New Triterpenes of the Fungus Ganoderma lucidum", Journal of Natural Products (1987); 50(5): 886-890.

50. Yasuo Komoda, Masato Shimizu, Yoshiko Sonoda and Yoshihiro Sato, "Ganoderic Acid and its Derivatives as Cholesterol Synthesis Inhibitors", Chemical and Pharmaceutical Bulletin (1989); 37(2): 531-533.

51. Aiko Morigiwa et. al., "Extraction of anti-hypertensive lanostane derivatives from mushrooms", (1987); in Chem. Abstr., CA107(6): 462752.

52. Hector O. Ventura and Franz H. Messerli, "Angiotensin-Converting Enzyme Inhibitors: A New Class of Antihypertensive Drugs". In Drug Therapy in Hypertension. Jan I.M. Drayer, David T. Lowenthal, and Michael A. Weber, editors. Marcel Dekker, Inc., 1987; 139-161.

53. John B. Kostis, M.D., Eugene A. De Felice, M.D. and Leonard J. Pianko, M.D., "The Renin-Angiotensin System". In Angiotensin Converting Enzyme Inhibitors. John B. Costis, M.D. and Eugene De Felice, M.D., editors. Alan R. Liss, Inc., 1987; 1-18.

54. Joe Graedon and Teresa Graedon. Joe Graedon's The New People Pharmacy: Drug Breakthroughs of the 80's. Bantam Books, 1985; 276-278.

55. Jack M. De Forrest, Thomas L. Waldron, Robert J. Scalese and Charlotte M. Harvey, "Biology of a novel class of potent long-acting angiotensin converting enzyme inhibitors: the acyl lys...... Journal of Hypertension (9188); 6(Suppl. 4): S470-S472.

56. Michinori Kubo, Hideaki Matsuda, Mari Nogami et al., "Studies on Ganoderma lucidum. IV. Effects on the Dissemenated Intravascular Coagulation", Yakugaku Zasshi (1983); 103(8): 871-877 (in Japanese).

57. Akira Shimizu, Takashi Yano, Yuji Saito and Yuji Inada, "Isolation of an Inhibitor of Platelet Aggregation from a Fungus, Ganoderma lucidum", Chemical and Pharmaceutical Bulletin (1985); 33(7): 3012-3015.

58. Harold A. Harper, Ph. D., Victor W. Rodwell, Ph. D., and Peter A. Mayes, Ph. D. Review of Physiologic Chemistry. Sixteenth edition. Lange Medical Publications, Los Altos, California, 1977; 109 and 297.

59. Ref. 54; 169-172.

60. Ref. 58; 261 and 458-459.

61. "adenosine 3': 5'-cyclic phosphote". Dorland's Illustrated Medical Dictionary. Twenty-sixth eiditon. W.B. Saunders, 1981; 32.126. Ref. 116; 127 and 219.

62. Ernest Lawrence Rossi. The Psychobiology of Mind-Body Healing. W.W. Norton, Inc., 1986; 112-113. (Italics added).

63. David Saphir, "Neurophysiological and Endocrine Consequences of Immune Activity", Psychoneuroimmunology (1989); 14(1/2): 63-87.

64. David F. Horrobin, "Essential Fatty Acids: A Review". In Clinical Uses of Fatty Acids. David F. Horrobin, editor. Eden Press, Inc., 1982; 3-36.

65. John Poppy, "The Chemistry of Love", Esquire, May 1989; 130-138.

66. Yoshimasa Kasahara and Hiroshi Hikino, "Central Actions of Adenosine, a Nucleotide ofGanoderma lucidum", Phytotherapy Research (1987); 1(4): 173-176.

67. Yoshimasa Kasahara and Hiroshi Hikino, "Central Actions of Ganoderma lucidum", Phytotherapy Research (1987); 1(1): 17-21.

68. Lee-Juian Lin, Ming-shi Shiao and Sheau-Farn Yeh, "Tripterpenes from Ganoderma lucidum", Phytochemistry (1988); 27(7): 2269-2271.

69. Eugene Feifel (trans.), "Pao-P'u Tzu Nei-P'ien, Chapter XI", Monumenta Serica (1946); 11; 1-32.

70. George F. Weber, "The Occurence of Tuckahoes and Poria cocos in Florida", Mycologia (1929); 21(3): 113-130.

71. Stephen Fulder, "Ginseng and the Hypothalamic-Pituitary Control of Stress", American Journal of Chinese Medicine (1981); 9(2): 112-118.

Notes for Chapters 5, 6 and 9

1. "Lingzhi". Pharmacology and Applications of Chinese Materia Medica, I. Hson-Mou Chang, Ph. D. and Paul Pui-Hay But, editors. World Scientific Publishing Co. Pte Ltd., Singapore, 1986; 642-653.

2. Product insert. Chung Wah Lingzhi Pian (Tabellae Ganodermatis). China Medicine and Health Product Import and Export Corporation, Hunan Branch, the People's Republic of China.

3. Tsutomu Tamura, Toshio Takahashi and Satoshi Matsuda, "Fermentation product as food for patients with mental diseases caused by environmental stresses", (1987); in Chem. Abstr. 108(13): 110851j.

4. Tsutomu Tamura, Toshio Takahashi and Satoshi Matsuda, "Fermentation product as food for patients with Alzheimer's disease", (1987); in Chem Abstr. 108(13): 110852k.

7. Fu Huidi and Wang Zhiyuan, "The Clinical Effects of Ganoderma lucidum Spore Preparations in 10 Cases of Atrophic Myotonia", Journal of Traditional Chinese Medicine (1982); 2(1): 63-65.

8. Zhang Juntien, "Recent Achievements of the Institute of Materia Medica on Studies of Natural Products". Proceedings of the U.S. China Pharmacology Symposium. J.J. Burns and P.J. Tsuchitani, editors. Washington, D.C., 1980; 15-54.

9. Jing-Guang Yu and Yun-Feng Zhai, "Studies on the Constituents of Ganoderma capens. Part I.", Yao Hsueh Hsueh Pao (1979); 14(6): 374-378, (in Chinese), in Chem. Abstr. 91: 181328k.

10. Geng-Tao Liu, Huai-Ling Wei, Tian-Tong Bao et al., "Effect of Ganodermas on elevated serum aldolase levels in experimental muscular dystrophy induced by 2,4-dichloro-phenoxyacetic acid (2,4-D) in mice", Yao Hsueh Hsueh Pao (1980); 15(3): 142-146, (in Chinese) in Chem. Abstr.;93: 179561d.

11. Jingguang Yu, Fushen Shen, Cuiying Hou and Shilin Yang, "Studies on chemical sonstituents of deep-layer fermentation mycelia of Ganoderma capense (Lloyd) Teng. Part II.", Zhongcaoyao (1981); 12(7): 7-11, (in Chinese), in Chem. Abstr. 96: 11554s.

12. Jingguang Yu, Ruoyun Chen and Zhixi Yao, "Studies on the chemical constituents of Bao Gai Ling Zhi (Ganoderma capense) mycelium by submerged fermentation. III.", Zhongcaoyao (1983); 14(10): 438-439, (in Chinese), in Chem. Abstr. 100: 66517p.

13. Guan de Zhang, Hong yue Liu and Yihon Liang, "Reverse-phase HPLC determination of nucleosides and their bases in the submerged culture of Ganoderma capense", Yaoxue Xuebao (1986); 21(1): 35-39, (in Chinese), in Chem Abstr. 104: 164583j. 14. D.M.O. Becroft and L.L. Phillips, "Hereditary Orotic Aciduria and Megaloblastic Anaemia: A Second Case, with Response to Uridine", British Medical Journal (1965); 1: 547-552.

15. "Uridine Triphosphate." Martindale: The Extra Pharmacopoeia. Twenty-eighth edition. E.F. Reynolds and Anne B. Prasad, editors. The Pharmaceutical Press, London, England, 1982; 1768.

16. Li-Hua Gao and Zhi-Yuan Wang, "The Inefficacy of Nucleic Acid Treatment in 9 Cases of Progressive Muscular Dystrophic Disease", Beijing Medical Journal (1981); 3(6): 347-348.

17. Fang Chu, Houliang Luo, Gui Luo et al., "Protection of nucleated bone marrow cells of mice against the effect of radiation-induced micronucleus formation with polysaccharides extracted from Zizhi (Ganoderma) ", Fushe Fanghu (1988); 8(1): 16-20, (in Chinese), in Chem. Abstr. 109(5): 34562u

18. Durk Pearson and Sandy Shaw. Life Extension. Warner Books, 1982; 182.

19. Sigeo Ukai, Tadashi Kiho, Chihiro Hara et al., "Polysaccharides in Fungi. XIV. Anti-inflammatory Effect of the Polysaccharides from the Fruit Bodies of Several Fungi", Journal of Pharmacobio-Dynamics (1983); 6(12): 983-990.

20. Wang Jifeng, Zhang Jiajun and Chen Wenwei, "Study of the Action of Ganoderma lucidum on scavenging hydroxyl Radical from Plasma", Journal of Traditional Chinese Medicine (1985); 5(1): 55-60. 21. Yao-Ren Dai, Chong-Ming Gao, Qing-Lai Tian and Ying Yin, "Effect of Extracts of Some Medicinal Plants on Superoxide Dismutase Activity in Mice", Planta Medica (1987); 53(3): 309-310.

22. Tsutomu Tamura, Toshio Takahashi and Satoshi Matsuda, "Fermentation product as food for patients with liver failure", (1987); in Chem. Abstr. 108(13): 110854n.

23. Liu Gengtao, Bao Tiantong, Niu Xinyi et al., "Some Pharmacological Actions of the Spores of Ganoderma lucidum and the Mycelium of Ganoderma capense (Lloyd) Teng. Cultivated by Submerged Fermentation", Chinese Medical Journal (1979); 92(7): 496-500.

24. S.H. Byun and I.H. Kim, "Studies on the Concurrent Administration of Medicines VIII. Effects of Concurrent Administration of Ganoderma lucidum Extract and Glutathione on the Liver Damage Induced by Carbon Tetrachloride in Rats", Journal of the Pharmaceutical Society of Korea (1987); 31(3): 133-139 (in Korean).

25. J. Kijima, J. Arai, S. Kusunoki and T. Furuya, "Establishing a D-Galactos-amine Induced Hepatic Injury Model using Primary Cultured Rat Hepatocytes", Soological Science (Tokyo) (1987); 4(6): 1000.

26. Geng-Tao Liu, Tian-Tong Bao, Huai-Ling Wei and .... "Some pharmacological effects of alcoholic extracts of Ganoderma lucidum and G. japonicum Lloyd on mouse liver", Yao Hsueh Hsueh Pao (1979); 14(5): 284-287, (in Chinese), in Chem. Abstr. 92: 51937t.

27. Geng-Tao Liu, Gui-Fen Wang, Huail-Ling Wei et al., "Comparison of the protective actions of dimethylbiphenyldicarboxylate, trans-stilbene, alcoholic extracts of Polyporus japonicus and Ganoderma towards experimental liver injury in mice", Yao Hsueh Hsueh Pao (1979); 14(10): 598-604, (in Chinese), in Chem. Abstr. 93: 542y.

28. Nanjing Branch of the National Medical Society, Association of Heart Vessels Disease and No. 6 Department of Hunan Institute of Pharmaceutical Industry. Clinical Observation on the Treatment of 103 Cases of Coronary heart Disease with Ganoderma Shu Xin Tablets, Chinese Traditional and Herbal Drugs (1979); (6): 32-33. Fu Kezhi, Trans.

29. The Third Hospital of Hong Qiao District in Tianjin. Clinical Observation on Hyperlipemia Treated with Linzhi (Ganoderma) tablets. Chinese Traditional and Herbal Drugs (1977); (1): 35-36. Fu Kezhi, Trans.

30. Subhuti Dharmananda, Chen Fu Tai, and George Weissmann, "Herbal Foods in Asia: Role in the Prevention and Treatment of Cardiovascular Diseases". In Nutrition and Heart Disease II. Ronald R. Watson, Ph. D., editor. CRC Press, Inc., Boca Raton, Florida, 1986; 96-97.

31. Katsuo Kanmatsuse, Nagao Kajiwara, Kyoko Hayashi et al., "Studies on Ganoderma lucidum. I. Efficacy against Hypertension and Side Effects", Yakugaku Zasshi (1985); 105(10): 942-947.

32. Liu Bo and Bau Yun-Sun. Fungi Pharmacopoeia (Sinica). the Kinoko Company, Oakland, California, 1980; 170-172.

33. Yoshimasa Kasahara and Hiroshi Hikino, "Central Actions of Ganoderma lucidum", Phytotherapy Research (1987); 1(1): 17-21.

34. S. Inoue and K. Honda, "Sleep-Promoting Effects of a Bracket Fungus, Fomes japonicus. " In Sleep '86. Eighth European Congress on Sleep Research, Szeged, Hungary, Sept. 1-5, 1986. W.P. Koella et al., editors. Gustav Fischer Verlag, Stuttgart, 1988; 338-339.

35. Masao Hirotani, Chieko Ino, Tsutomo Furuya and Motoo Shiro, "Ganoderic Acids T, S and R, New Triterpenoids from the Cultured Mycelia of Ganoderma lucidum", Chemical and Pharmaceutical Bulletin (1986); 34(5): 2282-2285.

36 Tsutomu Furuya, Yumiko Tsuda, Naoichi Koga et al., "Isolation of ganodosterone and ganoderic acids as liver function stimulants", in Chem. Abstr. 109(18): 156253q.

37. T. Tasaka, M. Mio, K. Izushi et al., "Anti-allergic constituents in the culture medium of Ganoderma lucidum. (II) The inhibitory effect of cyclooctasulpher on histamine release". Agents and Actions (1988); 23(3/4): 157-160.

38. Masaaki Ito et al., "Anti-allergic Effects of Reishi Ganoderma lucidum". Poster 24. International Congress on natural Products Research. American Society of Pharmacognosy and Japanese Society of Pharmacognosy. Twenty-ninth Annual Meeting of the American Society of Pharmacognosy, Park City, Utah, July 17-21, 1988. University of Utah, Dept. of Medicinal Chemistry, Salt Lake City, Utah, 1988.

40. Ian R. Tizzard. Immunology: An Introduction. Saunders College Publishing, Philadelphia, 1984; 352-365.

41. Mari Nogami, Yukiko Tsuji, Michinori Kubo et al., "Studies on Ganoderma lucidum. VI. Anti-allergic Effect. (1)", Yakugaku Zasshi (1986); 106(7): 594-599.

42. Mari Nogami, Masaaki Ito, Michinori Kubo et al., "Studies on Ganoderma lucidum. VII. Anti-allergic Effect. (2)", Yakugaku Zasshi (1986); 106(7): 600-604.

43. Ref. 40; 383.

44. Hiroshi Kohda, Wakao Tokumoto, Kiyoe Sakamoto et al., "The Biologically Active Constituents of Ganoderma lucidum (Fr.) Karst. Histamine Release-Inhibitory Triterpenes", Chemical and Pharmaceutical Bulletin (1985); 33(4): 1367-1374. Note: Ganoderic acid C was later renamed "C2".45

46. Aiko Morigawa, Katsuaki Kitabatake, Yoshinori Fujimoto and Nobue Ikekawa, "Angiotensin Converting Enzyme-Inhibitory Triterpenes from Ganoderma lucidum", Chemical and Pharmaceutical Bulletin (1986); 34(7): 3025-3028.

47. Ref. 40; 72.

48. Ref. 40; 120.

49. Ref. 40; 381-385.*

50. Ref. 40; 400-401.51. Ref. 40; 389-392.

52. Becoming Healthy With Reishi, III. Kampo I-yaku Shimbun, Toyo-Igaku Sha Co. Ltd., Tokyo, 1988; 12-20. Trans.

53. Ref. 40; 93-95.

54. Ref. 40; 322

55. Ref. 40; 95-97.

56. Ref. 40; 85.

57. Ref. 40; 267.

58. Bruce W. Halstead and Loretta L. Hood, "Natural Methods to Enhance Immunity", Bulletin of the Oriental Healing Arts Institute of U.S.A. (1984); 9(8): 377.

59. T. Tasaka, M. Akagi, K. Miyoshi et al., "Anti-allergic constituents in the culture medium of Ganoderma lucidum. (I) Inhibitory effect of oleic acid on histamine release", Agents and Actions (1988); 23 (3/4): 153-156.

60. Kohsuke Kino, Akio Yamashita, Kyoko Yamaoka et al., "Isolation and Characterization of a New Immunomodulatory Protein, Ling Zhi-8 (LZ-8), from Ganoderma lucidum ", The Journal of Biological Chemistry (1989); 264(1): 472-478.

61. Hiroshi Hikino, Chohachi Konno, Yoshiaki Mirin and Teruaki Hayashi, "Isolation and Hypoglycemic Activity of Ganoderans A and B, Glycans of Ganoderma lucidum Fruit Bodies", Planta Medica (1985); 51(3): 339-340.

62. Masashi Tomoda, Ryoko Gondo, Yoshimasa Kasahara and Hiroshi Hikino, "Glycan Structures of Ganoderans B and C, Hypoglycemic Glycans of Ganoderma lucidum Fruit Bodies", Phytochemistry (1986); 25(12): 2817-2820.

63. Yoshiyuki Kimura, Hiromichi Okuda and Shigeru Arichi, "Effects of the Extracts of Ganoderma lucidum on Blood Glucose Levels in Rats", Planta Medica (1988); 54(4): 290-294.

64. Tsutomu Tamura , Toshio Takahashi and Satoshi Matsuda, "Fermentation product as food for patients with diabetes", in Chem Abstr. (1987); 108(13): 110855p.

65. No. 201 Research Group of Hunan Institute of Pharmaceutical Industry. A Spot Survey on the Prevention of Acute Unadapted Symptoms at Plateau with Ganoderma. Chinese Traditional and Herbal Drugs (1979); (6): 29-31. Fu Kezhi, Trans.

66. M.J. Kim, H.W. Kim, Y.S. Lee et al., "Studies on Safety of Ganoderma lucidum", Korean Journal of Mycology (1986); 14(1): 49-60.

67. Subhuti Dharmananda, "Medicinal Mushrooms", Bestways Magazine, July, 1988.

68. Ewan Cameron and Linus Pauling, "Supplemental ascorbate in the supporative treatment of cancer: Prolongation of survival times in terminal human cancer", Proceedings of

the National Academy of Sciences U.S.A., (1976); 73(10): 3685-3689.

69. Akira Muratoa, Hiraku Suenaga, Shigetaka Hideshima et al., "Hydroxyl Radical as the Reactive Species in the Inactivation of Phages by Ascorbic Acid", Agricultural and Biological Chemistry (1986); 50(6): 1481-1487.

70. Robert F. Cathcart, III, "Vitamin C in the Treatment of Acquired Immune Deficiency Syndrome (AIDS)", Medical Hypotheses (1984); 14: 423-433.

‾ ‾ ‾ ‾ ‾ ‾ ‾otto ii_The Mysterious Reishi Mushroom. Woodbridge Press Publishing Company, Santa Barbara, California, 1979, ~~ ~~.

Notes for Chemical Chart in Appendices

1. T. Tasaka, M. Mio, K. Izushi et al., "Anti-allergic constituents in the culture medium of Ganoderma lucidum. II. The inhibitory effect of cyclooctasulpher [sic] on histamine release," Agents and Actions (1988); 23(3/4): 157-160.

2. "Lingzhi." Pharmacology and Applications of Chinese Materia Medica, I. Hson-Mou Chang, Ph.D. and Paul Pui-Hay But, editors. World Scientific Publishing Co. Pte Ltd., Singapore, 1986; 642-653.

3. Teikoku Chemical Industry Co., Ltd. Mushroom Glycoproteins as Neoplasm Inhibitors. Japanese Patent No. 82 75,926, May 12, 1982; in Chem. Abstr. 97: 44311j.

4. Martyna Kanderfer-Szersen, Zbigniew Kanecki and Maria Guz, "Fungal Nucleic Acids as Interferon Inducers," Acta Microbiologica (1979); 28(4): 277-291.

5. Zhang Juntien, "Recent Achievements of the Institute of Materia Medica on Studies of Natural Products." Proceedings of the U.S. China Pharmacology Symposium. J.J. Burns and P.J. Tsuchitani, editors. Washington, D.C., 1980; 15-54.

6. Jingguang Yu, Fuzhen Shen, Cuiying Hou and Shilin Yang, "Studies on chemical constituents of deep-layer fermentation mycelia of Ganoderma capense (Lloyd) Teng. Part II." Zhongcaoyao (1981); 12(7): 7-11 (in Chinese), in Chem. Abstr. 96: 11554s.

7. Li-Hua Gao and Zhi-Yuan Wang, "The Inefficacy of Nucleic Acid Treatment in 9 Cases of Progressive Muscular Dystrophic Disease," Beijing Medical Journal (1981); 3(6): 347-348.

8. Akira Shimizu, Takashi Yano, Yuji Sato and Yuji Inada, "Isolation of an Inhibitor of Platelet Aggregation from a Fungus, Ganoderma lucidum," Chemical and Pharmaceutical Bulletin (1985); 33(7): 3012-3015.

9. Yoshimasa Kasahara and Hiroshi Hikino, "Central Actions of Adenosine, a Nucleotide of Ganoderma lucidum," Phytotherapy Research (1987); 1(4): 173-176.

10. Hiroshi Hikino, Chohachi Konna, Yoshiaki Mirin and Teruaki Hayashi, "Isolation and Hypoglycemic Activity of Ganoderans A and B, Glycans of Ganoderma lucidum Fruit Bodies," Planta Medica (1985); 51(3): 339-340.

11. Masashi Tomoda, Ryoko Gondo, Yoshimasa Kasahara and Hiroshi Hikino, "Glycan Structures of Ganoderans B and C, Hypoglycemic Glycans of Ganoderma lucidum Fruit Bodies," Phytotherapy (1986); 25(12): 2817-2820.

12. Sigeo Ukai, Tadashi Kiho, Chihiro Hara et al., "Polysaccharides in Fungi. XIV. Anti-inflammatory Effect of the Polysaccharides from the Fruit Bodies of Several Fungi," Journal of Pharmacobio-Dynamics (1983); 6(12): 983-990.

13. Hitoshi Ito, Sensuke Naruse and Keishiro Shimura, "Studies on Antitumor Activity of Basidiomycete Polysaccharides. VII. Antitumor Effect of the Polysaccharide Preparations from Ganoderma lucidum on Mouse Sarcoma 180," Mie Medical Journal (1977); 26(2/3): 147-152.

14. Yoshiaki Sone, Reiko Okuda, Noriko Wada et al., "Structures and Antitumor Activities of the Polysaccharides Isolated from Fruiting Body and the Growing Culture of Mycelium of *Ganoderma lucidum,*" *Agricultural and Biological Chemistry* (1985); 49(9): 2641-2653.

15. Toshio Miyazaki and Motohiro Nishijima, "Studies on Fungal Polysaccharides. XXVII. Structural Examination of a Water-Soluble, Antitumor Polysaccharide of *Ganoderma lucidum,*" *Chemical and Pharmaceutical Bulletin* (1981); 29(12): 3611-3616.

16. Takuma Sasaki, Yoshiko Arai, Tetsuro Ikekawa, "Antitumor Polysaccharides from Some Polyporaceae, *Ganoderma applanatum* (Pers.) Pat. and *Phellinus linteus* (Berk. and Curt.) Aoshima," *Chemical and Pharmaceutical Bulletin* (1971); 19(4): 821-826.

17. Takashi Mizuno, Taichi Usui, Masashi Tomoda et al., "Studies on the Host-Mediated Antitumor Polysaccharides. II. Screening Test on Antitumor Activity of Various Kinds of Polysaccharides," *Shizuoka Daigaku Nogakubu Kenkyu Hokuku* (1980); (30): 41-50 (in Japanese), in *Chem. Abstr.* 94: 202749c.

18. Taichi Usui, Yoshio Iwasaki, Katsuyuki Hayashi et al., "Antitumor Activity of Water-Soluble Beta-D-Glucan Elaborated by *Ganoderma applanatum,*" *Agricultural and Biological Chemistry* (1981); 45(1): 323-326.

19. Takashi Mizuno, Naomi Kato, Atsushi Totsuka et al., "Fractionation, Structural Features and Antitumor Activity of Water-soluble Polysaccharide from "Reishi," the Fruit Body of *Ganoderm lucidum,*" *Nippon Nogei Kagaku Kaishi* (1984); 58(9): 871-880 (in Japanese), in *Chem. Abstr.* 101: 226886j.

20. Kureha Chemical Industry Co. Ltd., *Anticarcinogen.* Japanese Patent No. 76 17,166, May 31, 1976; in *Chem. Abstr.* 85: 190736v.

21. Hong Chang Guan and Zheng Cong, "Effects of Ling zhi polysaccharide D6 on the biosynthesis of nucleic acid protein and its preliminary analysis," *Yaoxue Tongbao* (1982); 17(3): 177-178 (in Chinese), in *Chem. Abstr.* 97: 155971u.

22. Kohsuke Kino, Akio Yamashita, Kyoko Yamaoka et al., "Isolation and Characterization of a New Immunomodulatory Protein, Ling Zhi-8 (LZ-8), from *Ganoderma lucidum,*" *The Journal of Biological Chemistry* (1989); 264(1): 472-478.

23. Tsutomu Furuya, Yumiko Tsuda, Naoichi Koga et al., "Isolation of ganodosterone and ganoderic acids as liver function stimulants," in *Chem. Abstr.* 109(18): 156253q.

24. Hiroshi Kohda, Wakao Tokumoto, Kiyoe Sakamoto et al., "The Biologically Active Constituents of *Ganoderma lucidum* (Fr.) Karst. Histamine Release-Inhibitory Triterpenes," *Chemical and Pharmaceutical Bulletin* (1985); 33(4); 1367-1374.

25. Masao Hirotani, Chieko Ino, Tsutomo Furuya and Motoo Shiro, "Ganoderic Acids T, S and R, New Triterpenoids from the Cultured Mycelia of *Ganoderma lucidum,*" *Chemical and Pharmaceutical Bulletin* (1986); 34(5): 2282-2285.

26. Akio Morigiwa, Katsuaki Kitabatake, Yoshinori Fujimoto and Nobuo Ikekawa, "Angiotension Converting Enzyme-Inhibitory Triterpenes from *Ganoderma lucidum,*" *Chemical and Pharmaceutical Bulletin* (1986); 34(7): 3025-3028.

27. Lee-Juian Lin, Ming-Shi Shiao and Sheu-Farn Yeh, "Triterpenes from *Ganoderma lucidum,*" *Phytochemistry* (1981); 27(7): 2269-2271.

28. Yasuo Komoda, Masato Shimizu, Yoshiko Sonoda and Yoshihiro Sato, "Ganoderic Acid and its Derivatives as Cholesterol Synthesis Inhibitors," *Chemical and Pharmaceutical Bulletin* (1989); 37(2): 531-533.

29. T. Tasaka, M. Akagi, K. Miyoshi et al., "Anti-allergic constituents in the culture medium of *Ganoderm lucidum.* (I). Inhibitory effect of oleic acid on histamine release," *Agents and Actions* (1988); 23(3/4): 153-156.

Index

A

B

161

V

W

X

Y

Z

About the Author

Terry Willard, Ph.D. has spent almost two decades studying the healing properties of the plant world. His books and courses are used throughout North America to teach aspiring herbalists the basic facts of their profession.

Dr. Willard has an extensive background in the research and design of herbal formulas. His "Wild Rose" products have been used for almost 15 years by people around the world. Terry is also a member of the Canadian Government's Expert Advisory Committee on Herbs and Botanical Preparations. As such he has been instrumental in the movement to legitimize and improve the use of herbs for health care.

Two previous books by Dr. Willard are in print. The first, *Healing Yourself with Natural Remedies (1984)*, is a general introduction to the use of natural remedies, ailment by ailment. The second, *Textbook of Modern Herbology (1988)*, is a first-year textbook for beginning herbalists. It reviews human anatomy and physiology, and describes the medicinal uses of major herbs.

Dr. Willard is also the founder of the Wild Rose College of Natural Healing which offers an extensive array of classroom and correspondence courses leading to diplomas in herbology and wholistic health therapy.

Terry practises in two natural health clinics, one in Calgary, Alberta, the other in Vancouver, British Columbia.

Those interested in acquiring Dr. Willard's books or requiring further information about his clinics or Wild Rose College are invited to contact:

Wild Rose College of Natural Healing
302, 1220 Kensington Rd. N.W.
Calgary, Alberta CANADA
T2N 3P5
(403) 270-0936